The Medical Effects of Nuclear War

The Medical Effects of Nuclear War

The Report of the British Medical Association's
Board of Science and Education

A Wiley Medical Publication

Published on behalf of the British Medical Association
by

JOHN WILEY & SONS
Chichester · New York · Brisbane · Toronto · Singapore

British Library Cataloguing in Publication Data:

British Medical Association. *(Board of Science
and Education)*

   The medical effects of nuclear war. — (a Wiley
medical publication)
   1. Atomic warfare.   2. Atomic bomb — physiological
effect
   I. Title

   616.9′897   RA646

   ISBN 0 471 90207 1

Phototypeset by Dobbie Typesetting Service, Plymouth, Devon
Printed by Page Brothers, Norwich

Contents

**Statement by the Council of the
    British Medical Association**   viii

Introduction   ix

Glossary   xv

Chapter 1   Physical principles and
    construction of nuclear weapons

Fission weapons   1
The physical effects of the Japanese explosions   3
Fusion weapons or thermonuclear weapons   6
Difference between air-burst and ground-burst explosions .   8
Evolution in guidance systems   9
The electromagnetic pulse (EMP)   12

Chapter 2   Nuclear attack on
    the United Kingdom

What form might a nuclear attack on the UK take?   15
National nuclear arsenals   16
Estimates of the possible scale of an attack   20
Ground-launched cruise missiles as targets   24
'Limited' attacks   25
The credibility of 'limited' nuclear war   26

Chapter 3   Mortality and morbidity
    consequent upon a nuclear attack

Part A   Injuries following a nuclear explosion   31
Radiation   33
Radiation sickness   33
The psychological effects   35

v

Treatment following a nuclear war   37
Medical response to infection in peacetime.   40
Destruction of medical facilities   40
Drugs   43

**Part B   Calculation of numbers of
casualties in a nuclear attack**   45

Casualty estimates for attacks on single cities or
  limited areas of the UK   48
Casualty estimates for attacks on the UK as a whole . . .   48
Discussion of uncertainties and variable factors in
  casualty estimates   56
Radiation levels from local fall-out.   71

**Implications of uncertainties and discrepancies
in assumptions for predicted casualties on
a national scale**   89

**Chapter 4   The long-term medical effects of
nuclear explosions**
Environmental health   92
Personal health 100

Chapter 5   Home defence
The present plan 106
Planning for emergencies 110

Chapter 6   The Health Service
Government assumptions in planning 112
DHSS responsibilities and medical plans for civil defence . 113
NHS wartime role 113
Role of voluntary organisations 116
Women's Royal Voluntary Service (WRVS) 116
Comments on current DHSS plans 119

Chapter 7   Summary and conclusions
Nuclear war affecting the United Kingdom 120
Civil Defence — Evacuation 121
Civil Defence — Shelters 122
Long-term effects of a nuclear attack 122
Effects on medical services 123

Annex 1 **Board of Science and Education terms of reference** 125

Annex 2 **Organisations and individuals who submitted evidence** 126

Annex 3 **Articles from the *British Medical Journal*** . . . 129

Annex 4 **Method of calculation of casualty numbers** . . 149

Annex 5 **Emergencies at nuclear reactor plants** 152

Annex 6 **Home Defence Circular HDC(77)1: The preparation and organisation of the Health Service for war** 155

References 176

Bibliography 179

Index 184

Statement by the Council of the British Medical Association

The Council wishes to express its thanks to the Board of Science and Education and to its Working Party under the Chairmanship of Sir John Stallworthy, for preparing this important report into the medical effects of nuclear war.

In submitting this report to the Representative Body the Council calls attention to the first sentence of the report—that its purpose is to provide an objective and scientific account of the medical consequences which would follow the explosion of nuclear weapons.

The report states that it was no part of the Working Party's terms of reference to consider the desirability or otherwise of stockpiling nuclear weapons and the Council therefore wishes to emphasise that its approval of publication of the report must not be interpreted as the expression by the Council of any view of the politics of nuclear armament or disarmament.

J. D. J. HAVARD
Secretary

Introduction

The purpose of this report is to give the reader an objective and scientific account of the medical consequences that would follow the explosion of nuclear weapons. Any statement made about the use of nuclear weapons is inevitably controversial and we have been acutely conscious of our responsibility to present objective findings.

On the basis of the information and evidence presented to us we have formed our judgements about the effects of nuclear war. Each reader must make personal decisions about matters connected with the nuclear weapons debate—including, for example, whether or not a home defence programme increases the likelihood of the event it is designed to mitigate. The desirability or otherwise of stockpiling a nuclear arsenal was not part of the terms of reference of this Working Party.

We began work on our inquiry into the medical effects of nuclear war in August 1981. At the end of this study, in February 1983, our knowledge of the effects of nuclear weapons is still far from perfect, but as we have learned more so our attitudes have evolved. It is difficult to compress the findings of that 18-month journey into a few thousand words. Nevertheless, we feel that the knowledge which we have gained has allowed us to produce a report containing much information of value to doctors and others concerned with these issues. Several of the organisations and individuals who co-operated in this inquiry had not previously considered aspects of their work from the medical standpoint.

Terms of reference

This report arose out of work done in accordance with a resolution passed by the 1981 Annual Representative Meeting (ARM) of the British Medical Association. Each division of the BMA, representing doctors in a geographical area, sends representatives to the ARM to debate issues that concern the practice of medicine and the common health. The ARM determines Association policy. In 1981 concern was expressed that members of the Association were being asked to participate in medical planning for the aftermath of a nuclear war at a time when the BMA had not formulated a policy based on a careful review of available scientific evidence.

After considering a composite motion aggregated from those submitted by several divisions, the ARM passed a resolution that:

The Board of Science and Education should review the medical effects of nuclear war and the value of civil defence in order that the British Medical Association should form a policy.

The Board of Science and Education agreed that a small working party should be set up to receive written and oral evidence from experts in many fields. The Working Party was constituted as follows:

Sir John Stallworthy	Emeritus Professor of Obstetrics and Gynaecology at the University of Oxford and past Chairman of the BMA's Board of Science and Education
Dr J. Stuart Horner	District Medical Officer of Croydon District Health Authority, and Chairman of the BMA's Central Committee for Community Medicine
Mr Kenneth McKeown CBE	Consultant Surgeon at Darlington Memorial Hospital and Member of the BMA's Board of Science and Education
Professor Peter Quilliam	Professor of Pharmacology at St Bartholomew's Hospital Medical College, London, and Chairman of the BMA's Board of Science and Education
Dr John Dawson	Under Secretary at the BMA, Head of the Professional Scientific and International Affairs Division

Secretaries: Miss R. Weston and subsequently Miss M. Barwood

The Board of Science and Education accepted the terms of reference for the inquiry suggested by the Working Party. A press statement set out the areas to be covered by the Working Party as follows:

1 The blast, thermal and immediate ionising radiation effects of nuclear weapons

2 The clinical problems, both immediate and delayed, likely to be caused by the detonation of nuclear weapons

3 Mortality and morbidity consequent upon varying nuclear attack patterns
4 Immediate and long-term psychiatric effects on survivors of a nuclear attack
5 The probable effects of a nuclear attack on the work, organisation, structure and management of the National Health Service
6 Relations between the National Health Service and organisations involved in civil defence.

Method of working

We decided that the medical effects of nuclear war should be examined sufficiently widely for the report to serve as a 'stand-alone' source of reference for doctors. The press statement invited written evidence, and a call was circulated for papers relevant to the inquiry. The organisations and individuals who gave written and oral evidence are listed in Annex 2.

Written evidence was studied carefully and a number of organisations and individuals were invited to meet the members of the Working Party to give supplementary information. Finally the Working Party drafted a report which was debated by the Board of Science and Education before being presented to the Council of the Association (written material was accepted for consideration up to February 1983).

Structure of the report

Chapter 1 starts by describing the construction of nuclear weapons and the events that occur in the course of a nuclear explosion. Nuclear weapons have many yields, sizes and designs, and the proportion of energy given off as blast, heat and radiation differs considerably from one to another. Casualty numbers and the short and long term physical damage vary considerably according to the type of weapon and the circumstances in which it is exploded. There have been substantial increases in the accuracy of weapon delivery systems in recent years modifying strategic planning and the possible medical effects of a nuclear war.

Chapter 2 of the report deals with the numbers and types of nuclear weapons in world arsenals and with the possible form of a nuclear attack on the United Kingdom. After the precision and relative accuracy of Chapter 1, the picture becomes much hazier when we examine possible scenarios for an attack on the UK using these weapons. Possible consequences of the deployment of cruise missiles in relation to the weight of a nuclear attack are examined and the credibility of the concept of 'limited' nuclear war is discussed.

Chapter 3 discusses the types of acute injuries caused by a nuclear attack and records our examination of the number of casualties that might be expected to follow an 'average' attack using nuclear weapons. We discuss the massive casualty figures expected from a single nuclear explosion and the facilities available to give presently acceptable methods of treatment to blast and trauma victims. It is clear from the evidence given to the Working Party that if we were involved in a nuclear war, we should be equipped with only the experience, drug stocks and health care facilities available in peacetime. This chapter also includes a detailed examination of the blast and damage figures which would result from an attack. Discrepancies between figures produced in Government publications and those of other authors were identified early in our discussions.

Chapter 4 deals with the long term medical effects of nuclear explosions. The essential requirements for some considerable time after an attack would be clean water, food in a form acceptable to humans, some shelter, power and fuel supplies. Medical services in their present form would be destroyed. A health service might not be re-established for some years following a nuclear attack on this country.

Chapter 5 deals with the existing plans produced by Government for home defence. It compares the plans that can be made for a major civilian disaster where fixed assumptions are possible, with the unknown situation following a nuclear attack. Higher levels of planning involving sophisticated coordination and management, successful in the Second World War, would be likely to break down following a nuclear attack. The problems attached to evacuation and to the provision of shelters are discussed.

Chapter 6 analyses Government's proposals for the National Health Service in time of war and sets out our comments.

Chapter 7 summarises the conclusions of the report.

Terminology

When radiation enters tissue, it loses energy. Alpha and beta particles, being charged, lose energy in electrical interactions with the atomic electrons near which they pass. Gamma rays and X-rays transfer energy in a variety of ways, but each involves the liberation of electrons, which then lose energy in electrical interactions. Neutrons also transfer energy in various ways, the most important being collisions with hydrogen nuclei, which are single protons; these protons are set in motion, and being charged, again lose energy in electrical interactions. In such electrical interactions, an electron may be ejected from an atom in a molecule, thus leaving the molecule positively charged.

The passage of a charged particle through atoms may also impart energy to the atomic electrons without actually ejecting them. This process is called excitation, which is dissipated as heat in tissue.

Ionising radiations cannot be directly detected by the human senses, but they can be detected and measured by a variety of means including photographic films, geiger tubes, and scintillation counters. Measurements made with such detectors can be interpreted in terms of the radiation dose absorbed by the body or by a particular part of the body. When measurements are not possible, as, for instance, when a radionuclide is deposited in an internal organ, it is possible to calculate the dose absorbed by that organ if the activity in it is known.

Absorbed dose is expressed in a unit called the gray, symbol Gy, after a British scientist (formerly expressed in a unit called the rad). It is a measure of the energy imparted by ionising radiation to a unit mass of matter such as tissue. A Gy corresponds to a joule per kilogram. Submultiples of the gray are frequently used, such as the centigray CGy, which equals one rad, and the microgray uGy.

Equal absorbed doses do not necessarily have equal biological effects: one Gy of alpha radiation to tissue, for instance, is more harmful than one Gy of beta radiation, because an alpha particle, being slower and more heavily charged, loses its energy much more densely along its path in tissue. To put all ionising radiations on an equal basis with regard to potential for causing harm, another quantity is needed. This is the dose equivalent. It is expressed in a unit named the sievert after a Swedish scientist, and its symbol is Sv. Dose equivalent is equal to the absorbed dose multiplied by a factor that takes account of the way a particular radiation distributes energy in tissue, thus influencing its effectiveness in causing harm. For gamma rays, X-rays, and beta particles, the factor is set at 1, and the gray and sievert are numerically equal. For alpha particles, the factor is 20, so that 1 Gy of alpha radiation corresponds to a dose equivalent of 20 Sv. Sub-multiples of the Sv are commonly used such as the millisievert, mSv.

Table 1. Relationship between old and new radiation units

	Old unit	Symbol	New unit	Symbol	Relationship
Activity	curie	Ci	becquerel	Bq	$1 \text{ Ci} = 3.7 \times 10^{10} \text{Bq}$
Absorbed dose	rad	rad	gray	Gy	$1 \text{ rad} = 0.01 \text{ Gy}$
Dose equivalent	rem	rem	sievert	Sv	$1 \text{ rem} = 0.01 \text{ Sv}$

Glossary

The glossary is placed at the front of the report because of the large number of technical terms unavoidably used in the text.

Absorbed dose. Quantity of ionising radiation. The amount of energy imparted to unit mass of matter such as tissue. Unit gray, symbol Gy .1 Gy = 1 joule per kilogram.

Actinides. A group of fifteen elements with atomic number from that of actinium (89) to lawrencium (103) inclusive. All are radioactive. Group includes uranium, plutonium, americium, curium.

Activity. Quantity of a radionuclide. Describes the rate at which decays occur in an amount of radionuclide. Unit becquerel, symbol Bq. One Bq corresponds to the decay of one radionuclide per second.

Advanced Gas-cooled Reactor (AGR). A development of the Magnox reactor, using enriched uranium oxide fuel in stainless steel containers.

Alpha particle. A particle consisting of two protons plus two neutrons, emitted spontaneously from the nuclei of some radioactive elements. It is identical with a helium nucleus, having a mass of four units and an electric charge of two positive units.

Atom. The smallest portion of an element that can combine chemically with other atoms.

Atom bomb. See nuclear weapon.

Atomic number. The number of protons in the nucleus of an atom. Symbol Z.

Becquerel. See activity.

Beta particle. A particle, emitted by a radionuclide, with mass and charge equal in magnitude to an electron. The electric charge may be positive, in which case, the beta particle is called a positron.

Cloud column. The visible column of weapon debris (and possibly dust and water droplets) extending upward from the point of burst of a nuclear (or atomic) weapon.

Collective dose. Frequently used for collective effective dose equivalent.

Collective effective dose equivalent. The quantity obtained by multiplying the average effective dose equivalent by the numbers of persons exposed to a given source of radiation. Expressed in man-sievert, symbol man-Sv. Frequently abbreviated to collective dose.

Crater. The pit, depression, or cavity formed in the surface of the Earth by a surface or underground explosion. Crater formation can occur by vaporisation of the surface material, by the scouring effect of air blast, by throwout of disturbed material, or by subsidence. In general, the way in which the crater is formed changes from one to the next with increasing depth of burst. The apparent crater is the depression which is seen after the burst. It is smaller than the true crater because it is covered with a layer of loose earth, rock etc.

Cosmic rays. High-energy ionising radiations from outer space.

Decay. The spontaneous transformation of a radionuclide. The decrease in the activity of a radioactive substance.

Decay product. A nuclide or radionuclide produced by decay. It may be formed directly from a radionuclide or as a result of a series of successive decays through several radionuclides.

Depleted uranium. Uranium in which the content of the isotope uranium-235 has been decreased. Refers to a decrease below the natural value of 0.7% by weight or to a decrease below the desired content in enriched uranium.

DNA. Deoxyribonucleic acid. The compound that controls the structure and function of cells and is the material of inheritance.

Dose. General term for quantity of radiation. See absorbed dose, dose equivalent, effective dose equivalent, collective effective dose equivalent. Frequently used for effective dose equivalent.

Dose equivalent. The quantity obtained by multiplying the absorbed dose by a factor to allow for the different effectiveness of the various ionising radiations in causing harm to tissue. Unit sievert, symbol Sv. The factor for gamma rays, X-rays, and beta particles is 1, for neutrons 10, and for alpha particles 20.

Dynamic pressure. The air pressure that results from the mass air flow (or wind) behind the shock front of a blast wave. It is equal to the product of half the density of the air through which the blast wave passes and the square of the particle (or wind) velocity behind the shock front as it impinges on the object or structure.

Effective dose equivalent. The quantity obtained by multiplying the dose equivalents to various tissues and organs by the risk weighting factor appropriate to each and summing the products. Expressed in sieverts, symbol Sv. Frequently abbreviated to dose.

Electrical interaction. A force of repulsion acting between electric charges of like sign and a force of attraction acting between electric charges of unlike sign.

Electromagnetic Pulse (EMP). A sharp pulse of radio frequency electromagnetic radiation produced when an explosion occurs in an unsymmetrical environment, especially at or near the Earth's surface or at high altitudes. The intense electric and magnetic fields can damage unprotected electrical and electronic equipment over a large area.

Electron. An elementary particle with low mass, 1/1836 that of a proton, and with unit negative electric charge. Positively-charged electrons, called positrons, also exist. See beta particle.

Electron volt. Unit of energy employed in radiation physics. Equivalent to the energy gained by an electron in passing through a potential difference of 1 volt. Symbol eV. $1eV = 1.6 \times 10^{-19}$ joule approximately.

Element. A substance with atoms all of the same atomic number.

Enriched uranium. Uranium in which the content of the isotope uranium-235 has been increased above its natural value of 0.7% by weight.

Excitation. A process by which radiation imparts energy to an atom or molecule without causing ionisation. Dissipated as heat in tissue.

Fall-out. The transfer of radionuclides produced by nuclear weapons from the atmosphere to Earth. The process or phenomenon of the descent to the Earth's surface of particles contaminated with radioactive material from the radioactive cloud. The term is also applied in a collective sense to the contaminated particulate matter itself. The early (or local) fall-out is defined, somewhat arbitrarily, as those particles which reach the Earth within 24 hours after a nuclear explosion. The delayed (or worldwide) fall-out consists of the smaller particles that ascend into the upper troposphere and into the stratosphere and are carried by winds to all parts of the Earth. The delayed fall-out is brought down to Earth, mainly by rain and snow, over extended periods ranging from months to years.

Fast neutrons. Conventionally, neutrons with energies in excess of 0.1 MeV. Corresponding velocity about 4×10^6 m s^{-1}.

Fast reactors. See nuclear reactor.

Fire storms. Stationary mass fire, generally in built-up urban areas, causing strong, inrushing winds from all sides; the winds keep the fires from spreading while adding fresh oxygen to increase their intensity.

Fission products. A general term for the complex mixture of substances produced as a result of nuclear fission. A distinction should be made between these and the direct fission products of fission fragments that are formed by the actual splitting of the heavy-element nuclei. Something like 80 different fission fragments result from roughly 40 different modes of fission of a given nuclear species (e.g., uranium-235 or plutonium-239). The fission fragments, being radioactive, immediately begin to decay, forming additional (daughter) products, with the result that the complex mixture of fission products so formed contains over 300 different isotopes of 36 elements.

Fission. Nuclear fission. A process in which a nucleus splits into two or more nuclei and energy is released. Frequently refers to the splitting of a nucleus of uranium-235 into two approximately equal parts by a thermal neutron with emission of other neutrons.

Free radical. A grouping of atoms that normally exists in combination with other atoms, but can sometimes exist independently. Generally very reactive in a chemical sense.

Fusion. Thermonuclear fusion. A process in which two or more light nuclei are formed into a heavier nucleus and energy is released.

Gamma rays (or radiations). Electromagnetic radiations of high photon energy, without mass or charge, propagated as a wave, originating in atomic nuclei and accompanying many nuclear reactions (e.g., fission, radioactivity, and neutron capture). Physically, gamma rays are identical with X-rays of high energy, the only essential difference being that X-rays do not originate from atomic nuclei but are produced in other ways (e.g. by slowing down (fast) electrons of high energy).

Geiger tube. A glass or metal envelope containing a gas at low pressure and two electrodes. Ionising radiation causes discharges, which are registered as electric pulses in a counter. The number of pulses is related to dose.

Height of Burst (HOB). The height above the Earth's surface at which a bomb is detonated in the air.

Kiloton energy. Defined strictly as 10^{12} calories (or 4.2×10^{19} ergs). This is approximately the amount of energy that would be released by the explosion of 1000 tons of TNT.

Magaton energy. Defined strictly as 10^{15} calories (or 4.2×10^{22} ergs). This is approximately the amount of energy that would be released by the explosion of 1000 kt (1 million tons) of TNT.

Molecule. The smallest portion of a substance that can exist by itself and retain the properties of the substance.

Mutation. A chemical change in the DNA in the nucleus of a cell. Mutations in sperm or egg cells or their precursors may lead to inherited effects in children. Mutations in body cells may lead to effects in the individual.

Neutron. A neutral particle (i.e., with no electrical charge) of approximately unit mass, present in all atomic nuclei, except those of ordinary (light) hydrogen. Neutrons are required to initiate the fission process, and large numbers of neutrons are produced by both fission and fusion reactions in nuclear (or atomic) explosions.

Nuclear power. Power obtained from the operation of a nuclear reactor. Refers in the text to electric power.

Nuclear radiation. Particulate and electromagnetic radiation emitted from atomic nuclei in various nuclear processes. The important nuclear radiations, from the weapons standpoint, are alpha and beta particles, gamma rays, and neutrons. All nuclear radiations are ionising radiations, but the reverse is not true. X-rays, for example, are included among ionising radiations, but they are not nuclear radiations since they do not originate from atomic nuclei.

Nuclear weapon (or bomb). A general name given to any weapon in which the explosion results from the energy released by reactions involving atomic nuclei, either fission or fusion, or both. Thus, the A- (or atomic) bomb and H- (or hydrogen) bomb are both nuclear weapons. It would be equally true to call them atomic weapons, since it is the energy of atomic nuclei that is involved in each case. However, it has become more or less customary, although it is not strictly accurate, to refer to weapons in which all the energy results from fission as A-bombs or atomic bombs.

Nuclear reactor. A device in which nuclear fission may be sustained in a self-supporting chain reaction involving neutrons. In thermal reactors, fission is brought about by thermal neutrons, in fast reactors by fast neutrons.

Nucleus. The core of an atom, occupying little of the volume, containing most of the mass, and bearing positive electric charge.

Nucleus of cell. The kernel of the basic unit of tissue. Contains the important material DNA.

Nuclide. A species of atom characterised by the number of protons and neutrons and, in some cases, by the energy state of the nucleus.

Order of magnitude. Quantity given to the nearest power of ten.

Proton. An elementary particle with approximately unit atomic mass and with unit positive electric charge.

PWR. Pressurised water reactor.

Radiation. The process of emitting energy as waves or particles. The energy thus radiated.

Radioactive. Possessing radioactivity.

Radioactivity. The property of radionuclides of spontaneously emitting ionising radiation. By extension, materials containing radionuclides.

Radiological protection. The science and practice of limiting the harm to humans from radiation.

Radionuclide. An unstable nuclide that emits ionising radiation.

Risk. The probability of injury, harm or damage.

Risk factor. The probability of cancer and leukaemia or hereditary damage per unit dose equivalent. Usually refers to fatal malignant diseases and serious hereditary damage. Symbol Sv^{-1}.

Sievert. See effective dose equivalent.

Sorption. In relation to the transport of radionuclides by ground-water through rock and soil, processes such as adsorption, ion exchange, precipitation, colloidal filtration, and mineralisation.

Teragram. 10^9 kilograms = one thousand million kilograms.

TNT. Trinitrotoluene—a conventional high explosive used as a standard measure of explosive power.

X-ray. A discrete quantity of energy, without mass or charge, that is propagated as a wave. See gamma ray.

CHAPTER 1

Physical principles and construction of nuclear weapons

This chapter traces the history of the development of nuclear weapons from 1945—when two fission weapons were exploded over Japan at Hiroshima and Nagasaki—to the present time. It includes a survey of the current range of nuclear weapons known to be in existence.

The physics and construction of nuclear weapons is described because it is impossible to appreciate the medical consequences of a nuclear war without some understanding of the processes involved.

It is also important to appreciate the changes brought about by developments in micro-electronics applied to the devices (the guidance systems) that steer nuclear weapons to their targets.

It is not enough simply to multiply the effects of the Japanese explosions in order to form a picture of the effects of a nuclear war on the United Kingdom.

Several small weapons released from a single missile cause more damage and casualties than a single warhead with equivalent yield delivered by the same missile.

Electronic communications systems are essential for effective health care. These systems can be disrupted or destroyed by the very strong electric field (the electromagnetic pulse or EMP) resulting from high altitude nuclear explosions.

Fission weapons

The basic nuclear weapon is the fission bomb. The weapon used against Hiroshima (code named 'Little Boy') was a free-fall bomb dropped from an aircraft at 8.15 am on 6 August 1945. The bomb exploded approximately 500 metres above the centre of the city with a force, or yield, said to be equivalent to approximately 12,500 tons (12.5 kilotons) of TNT. The explosion was several thousand times more powerful than that produced by any previous conventional bomb.

The bomb used to destroy Nagasaki (code named 'Fat Man') exploded 500 metres above the city at 11.02 am on 9 August 1945. It is thought to have had an explosive yield of some 22 kilotons. 'Fat Man' was about three metres long, 1.5 metres wide, and weighed 4,500 kilograms.

In these A-bombs, as they were called, a fission chain reaction was triggered and sustained in order to produce a very large amount of energy in a very short time. Within a millionth of a second the effect of heat on the surrounding air and objects created a very powerful explosion.

The atomic bombs built so far have used uranium-235 or plutonium-239 as the fissile material. A fission event occurs when a neutron enters the nucleus of an atom of one of these materials, which then breaks up or 'fissions'. A large amount of energy is released, the original nucleus is split into two radioactive nuclei (the fission products) and two or three neutrons are released. These neutrons can be used to produce a self-sustaining chain reaction. A chain reaction will take place only if at least one of the neutrons released in each fission produces a fission reaction in another heavy nucleus.

The smallest amount of the material in which a self-sustaining chain reaction (and hence a nuclear explosion) will take place is the critical mass. The critical mass depends on the nuclear properties of the material used for the fission, for instance, uranium-235 or plutonium-239. The higher the density of the material the shorter the average distance travelled by a neutron before causing another fission, and, therefore, the smaller the critical mass.

If the material is impure some neutrons may be captured by the nuclei of the non-fissile contaminants instead of causing fission. If the material is surrounded by a medium like natural uranium, which reflects neutrons back into the 'core' material, some neutrons may be used for fission which would otherwise have been lost. This method of construction will reduce the critical mass.

The critical mass of, for example, a bare sphere of pure plutonium-239 metal in its densest phase would be approximately 10 kilograms (22 pounds), about the size of a small grapefruit. If the sphere were surrounded by a natural uranium neutron reflector the critical mass would be reduced to about 4.4 kilograms (10 pounds). This would amount to a sphere of about 3.6 centimetres (1.4 inches) in radius— about the size of an orange. Using a technique called implosion, in which conventional explosive lenses are used to compress a mass which is slightly less than critical to a mass which is slightly greater than critical, a nuclear explosion could be achieved with less than 2 kilograms

(4.4 pounds) of plutonium-239. A 2-kilogram sphere of plutonium-239 would have a radius of about 2.8 centimetres (1.1 inches), making it smaller than a tennis ball.

In a nuclear explosion there is a very rapid build up of extremely high temperatures (hundreds of millions of degrees Centigrade) and very high pressures (millions of atmospheres). The chain reaction reaches a climax in about half a millionth of a second, the time taken for about 55 generations of fission. The mass of the fissile material expands at very high speeds, initially at a speed of about 1000 kilometres (652 miles) per second.

In much less than a millionth of a second the size and density of the fissile material have changed so that the mass becomes less than critical and the chain reaction stops. A nuclear weapon can only explode if the fissile material is kept together, against its tendency to fly apart, long enough to get sufficient generations of fission.

Two different mechanisms were used to detonate the nuclear weapons dropped over Japan. In the Hiroshima bomb, a sub-critical mass of uranium-235 was fired down a 'gun' into another sub-critical mass placed in front of the 'muzzle'. When these two masses came together they formed a super-critical mass which exploded. About 60 kilograms (132 pounds) of uranium-235 were used in the Hiroshima bomb, of which about 700 grams (1.5 pounds) were fissioned. The average time between spontaneous fissions was about one-fiftieth of a second, adequate for the 'gun' technique.

In the Nagasaki bomb the plutonium-239 core was surrounded by chemical explosives arranged as explosive lenses focused on the centre of the plutonium sphere. When these lenses were detonated the sphere was compressed uniformly by the implosion. The compression increased the density of the plutonium core so that the sub-critical mass was made super-critical. The complete detonation of 1 kilogram (2.2 pounds) of plutonium would produce an explosion equivalent to that of 18 kilotons of TNT. The eight kilograms of plutonium in the Nagasaki bomb produced an explosion equivalent to that of 22 kilotons of TNT. Its efficiency, therefore, was only about 15 per cent.

The physical effects of the Japanese explosions

Hiroshima is built on a plateau and, consequently, the city was damaged symmetrically in all directions. The damage to Nagasaki, built on mountainous ground, varied considerably according to the terrain in each direction. But the death rate at given distances from ground zero (the point on the ground directly below the centre of the explosion) was about the same in both cities.

Almost everyone within 500 metres of ground zero when the bombs exploded was killed; about 60 per cent of those within 2 kilometres died. About three-quarters of these deaths occurred in the first 24 hours.

The number of people in Hiroshima at the time of the bomb is not clear. The best estimate is that about 350,000 people were in the city. At the beginning of November 1945, 130,000 of these people or approximately 40 per cent of the population of Hiroshima had died, but even this high figure is almost certainly an underestimate. Many thousands of people were found to be unaccounted for in the 1950 National Census. The number that initially survived but died in the next few years is unknown; so too is the fate of the very large number of people who entered Hiroshima within the first week of the bombing.

About 270,000 people, including many Koreans, are thought to have been in Nagasaki when the bomb exploded. According to the best estimate some 60–70,000 died by the end of 1945. The number of Nagasaki A-bomb victims who died after 1945 is not known.

These 'best estimates' for casualties in the Japanese bombings are from the most recent and comprehensive study, in which all available sources of data have been reviewed and re-evaluated[1]. Much lower totals of deaths and injuries have been reported in the past, and been given wide prominence, particularly in American publications[2]; but those figures have now been effectively superseded. Most of the discrepancies are accounted for not so much through disagreement about the physical effects of the weapons, but because of widely differing estimates of the numbers of people who were actually present in the two cities on the dates of the attacks. Most authorities, Japanese, American and British, agree quite closely on the *percentages* of the population present who were killed and injured at different distances from the explosions.

Of those killed immediately, most were either crushed or burned to death. The combined effect of thermal radiation and blast was particularly lethal. Many of those burned to death in collapsed buildings would have escaped with only minor injuries had there been no fires. However, an area of 13 square kilometres in Hiroshima and 7 square kilometres in Nagasaki was reduced to rubble by blast and then to ashes by fire. The difference in size of these two devastated areas was due mainly to variations in the topography.

About half of the energy generated by the atomic bombs was given off as blast (see Figure 1.1). The front of the blast moved as a shock wave — a wall of high-pressure air, spreading outward at a speed equal to or greater than that of sound—covering about 11 kilometres in 30 seconds.

The shock wave was followed by a hurricane-force wind. As the shock wave travelled outward, it left behind an area of negative pressure, and eventually the air flowed in the inward direction. Thus, a supersonic shock wave was followed by an overpowering wind and then after an instant of stillness, a violent wind blew back in the opposite direction.

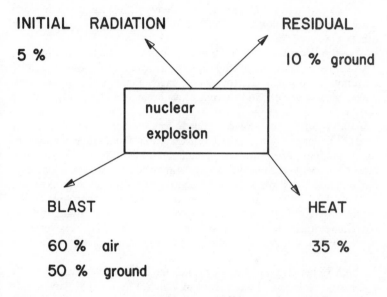

Figure 1.1. This illustration relates to a ground-burst. In an air-burst the blast is increased by 10% to form 60% of the total and there is a greatly diminished residual radiation component

At Hiroshima all buildings within two kilometres of ground zero were damaged beyond repair by overpressures (pressures in excess of atmospheric pressure) of 4 pounds per square inch (psi) and greater. Casualties due to blast were particularly severe within about 1.3 kilometres of ground zero, where the overpressures reached levels of 10 psi and greater.

About one-third of the total energy generated by the bombs was given off as heat. The fireballs produced by the nuclear explosions reached temperatures of the same magnitude as that of the sun almost instantly.

The fireballs grew to their maximum diameters of about 400 metres within a second, when their surface temperatures were about 5000°C.

At a distance of 500 metres from ground zero in Hiroshima the thermal radiation received in the first three seconds was about 600 times as great as the sun on a bright day. Even at a distance of 3 kilometres from the ground zero, the heat in the first 3 seconds was about 40 times more than that from the sun. The heat at Nagasaki was more intense, twice that at Hiroshima.

The heat was sufficient to burn exposed human skin at distances as great as 4 kilometres from ground zero. Many people caught in the open within about 1.2 kilometres from ground zero were burned to death; others were vaporised.

Hiroshima had about 76,000 buildings before the bomb was dropped. Two-thirds were destroyed by fire. A quarter of Nagasaki's 51,000 buildings were totally destroyed, and many more seriously damaged. The extensive damage and absence of water made effective fire-fighting impossible.

In both cities people were exposed to radiation of three different kinds. The largest dose was from direct initial radiation at the time of the detonation. The estimates of radiation doses from this source have recently undergone revision and are still subject to some controversy. Some radioactivity was induced by neutrons resulting in some exposure to those who entered the area around ground zero shortly after the explosion. Since both the weapons were air-burst, local fall-out did not contribute greatly to exposure although at Nagasaki one area received moderate doses of radiation due to rain which precipitated some fall-out.

About 15 per cent of the energy generated by the bombs was given off as ionising radiation, about a third of which, the initial radiation, was emitted within 1 minute of the explosion. The remainder, the residual radiation, was emitted from radioactive material in the form of 'fall-out'. The initial radiation dose at ground zero in Hiroshima was of the order of 1000 grays (100,000 rads). In Nagasaki the dose at this point was several times greater.

Fusion weapons or thermonuclear weapons

The maximum explosive yield achievable by pure fission weapons is limited by the critical mass to a few tens of kilotons. The next significant advance in warhead design after the Nagasaki bomb was the 'boosted weapon' in which fusion was used to obtain nuclear explosions with yields in the 100,000 ton (100-kiloton) range.

Fusion reaction is the opposite of fission. In fusion, light nuclei are formed (fused) into heavier ones; isotopes of hydrogen — deuterium and tritium — are fused together to form helium. The reaction produces very large quantities of energy and is accompanied by the emission of neutrons. There is no critical mass for the fusion process and therefore in principle there is no limit to the explosive yield of fusion weapons or H-bombs.

A fission reaction is relatively easy to start — one neutron will initiate a chain reaction in a critical mass of fissile material. But fusion is possible only if the component positively charged nuclei are given a high enough energy to overcome the repulsive electric force between them. In the H-bomb this energy is provided by raising the temperature of the fusion material. H-bombs, therefore, are also called thermonuclear weapons.

Professor J Rotblat has described the technique used thus[3]:

The solution to the problem lies in the fact that at the very high temperature of the fission trigger most of the energy is emitted in the form of X-rays. These X-rays travelling with the speed of light, radiate out from the center and on reaching the tamper (surrounding the fusion material) are absorbed in it and then immediately re-emitted in the form of softer X-rays. By an appropriate configuration of the trigger and the fusion material it is possible to ensure that the X-rays reach the latter almost instantaneously. If the fusion material is subdivided into small portions, each surrounded with a thin absorber made of a heavy metal, the bulk of the fusion material will simultaneously receive enough energy to start the thermonuclear reaction before the explosion disperses the whole assembly.

In order to make the deuterium-tritium fusion reaction work, a temperature of a hundred million degrees Centigrade or so is required. This can be provided only by an A-bomb in which such a temperature is achieved at the moment of the explosion. An H-bomb, therefore, consists of a fission stage, which is an A-bomb acting as a trigger, and a fusion stage, in which hydrogen is ignited by the heat produced by the trigger.

H-bombs are much more difficult to design than A-bombs. The problem is to prevent the A-bomb trigger from blowing the whole weapon apart before the fusion reaction has proceeded far enough to give the required explosive yield. Sufficient energy has to be delivered to the fusion material to start the thermonuclear reaction in a time much shorter than the time it takes for the explosion to occur. This requires that the energy be delivered with a speed approaching the speed of light. It is this requirement that makes the design of an H-bomb much more sophisticated than that of an A-bomb.

The energy released from an H-bomb comes from the fission trigger and the fusion material. But if the fusion weapon is surrounded by a shell of uranium-238 the high energy neutrons produced in the fusion process will cause additional fissions in the uranium shell. This technique can be used to enhance considerably the explosive power of an H-bomb. Such a weapon is called a fission-fusion-fission device. On average, about half of the yield from a typical thermonuclear weapon will come from fission and the other half from fusion.

Although designs based on the Hiroshima and Nagasaki bombs might still be used by countries beginning a nuclear weapon program, they are crude compared with current American and Soviet nuclear warheads. In comparison to the Nagasaki bomb, a typical modern American warhead weighs about 100 kilograms (220 pounds) and has an explosive power of about 350 kilotons of TNT. The yield-to-weight ratio, the standard measure of the efficiency of a bomb, has advanced from about 5000 for the Nagasaki bomb to about 3.5 million for today's best nuclear warheads. The latter figure is, in fact, close to the theoretical maximum attainable. Another indication of the sophistication of modern nuclear warheads is that they can be fitted into 8-inch artillery shells and made light enough (approximately 40 kgs) to be fired long distances.

Very large yields have been obtained in fusion weapons. In 1962, the Soviet Union exploded an H-bomb with a yield equal to that of 58 million tons of TNT equivalent (58 megatons), roughly the equal of 3000 Nagasaki bombs. Even higher yields could be obtained. Such huge bombs, however, make little sense. The largest city would be completely demolished by an H-bomb of 10 megatons or so.

Differences between air-burst and ground-burst explosions

The physical effects of a given weapon will vary according to a number of factors. An important variable is the height above ground at which the bomb is detonated. If this height is such that the resulting fireball touches the ground, it is said to be a 'ground-burst'. For any height above this, it is an 'air-burst'.

The range of blast effects will be greater for an air-burst than for an equivalent yield ground-burst. The principal reason is that the shock wave from the explosion is reflected from the ground and combines with the direct wave to produce a merged or Mach wave. Thus a military planner wishing to cause the maximum damage to unprotected targets such as cities or large industrial areas, would tend to employ air-burst weapons. Both of the bombs used in Japan were air-burst. It is possible to 'optimise' the height of detonation so as to subject the greatest possible area to a chosen level of blast overpressure.

With a ground-burst bomb on the other hand, much higher levels of blast pressure can be created at ground zero. A proportion of the energy of the bomb will be transmitted into the ground, producing not only a crater but also a spreading 'earthquake' effect that can seriously damage underground structures such as sewers, water pipes, and electricity supply cables. This is the second reason why the range of blast effects is reduced by comparison with an air-burst. The obstructions presented by buildings and hills can also limit the range of thermal and nuclear radiation from a ground-burst.

So far as casualties go, the process of formation of the crater is not of interest as such since within this range the destruction will be total and casualties 100 per cent. However, the vast quantities of dirt and debris gouged out of the crater are sucked up into the fireball, and it is these radioactive materials which are later deposited as fall-out. By comparison the quantities of fall-out created by an air-burst are very small.

Some of the fall-out, the larger particles, will return to earth within hours or days. This is 'early fall-out'. Meanwhile the smaller particles may be carried up into the stratosphere, where they can remain for months or even years before falling slowly to the ground again. This is 'delayed fall-out'; it may be dispersed on a global scale. With ground-burst explosions about 40 per cent of the fall-out remains air-borne for long periods.

The early fall-out is deposited on the areas immediately around and down-wind from the explosion, over distances which can extend to hundreds of kilometres, in a complex pattern which is difficult to predict with accuracy. Much of what is known about the behaviour of fall-out clouds comes from the monitoring of American atmospheric tests in the Pacific in the 1950s.

Evolution in guidance systems

The components of nuclear weapons have evolved continually since 1945. According to a 1981 report from the United Nations Centre for Disarmament[4]:

Rockets may carry one or several warheads, which may be independently targeted. The multiple independently targetable re-entry vehicle (MIRV) system was developed by the United States in the late 1960s and is deployed also by the Soviet Union. In a MIRVed system, the separate re-entry vehicles are

usually carried on a 'bus' which releases the RVs one by one after making pre-
selected changes in speed and orientation so as to direct the RVs to their
separate targets. These RVs can reportedly land inside an area of perhaps
150 km by 500 km. Thus, they are not as completely independent in arrival time
or location as they would be were they on different ICBMs, and they provide
less targeting flexibility.

With increasing missile accuracy and many RVs per missile, MIRV has raised
the spectre that a fraction of one side's ICBM forces may in a 'first strike'
destroy the opponent's ICBMs still housed in their hardened silos. This
situation is therefore considered to be potentially unstable, since in time of crisis
each side may consider launching its missiles rather than risking their
destruction.

If a target is vulnerable to a particular pressure level of air blast, its destruction
may be achieved within a certain maximum area around the point of detonation.
The size of this area increases with the weapon yield (e.g., by a factor 4 for an
8-fold increase in yield or a factor 100 for a 1000-fold increase in yield). By
contrast, the area of destruction due to blast increases in proportion to the
number of weapons (Figure 1.2). This means in practice that the destruction is
increased by increasing the number of warheads and lowering their individual
RV yield; i.e. one large warhead is not so effective as several smaller ones of the
same total yield spread out over the target area.

Guidance systems for vehicles (and for some types of mobile platforms) are of
particular interest. Here it is necessary to distinguish between ballistic missiles,
which are guided mainly during the 'boosting' phase, i.e., the initial part of the
flight when the rocket engines work; vehicles like cruise missiles, which are
driven through the entire flight path and for which guidance becomes
navigation; and weapons (of any kind) in their final approach to the target, when
target-finding and homing devices developed for conventional munitions might
be used.

For homing a weapon on the target, a number of sensors have been developed
to govern the operations of steering mechanisms in the projectile. These homing
systems include a variety of radar, infrared and laser devices. Some of them
could be adapted for use within strategic vehicles; others may be used to
enhance the accuracy of various tactical nuclear weapons. To what extent the
nuclear-weapon states have already implemented such options is not known,
although nuclear-weapon states have not deployed guidance systems for re-entry
vehicles from ballistic missiles.

The lethality of nuclear weapons has steadily (Figure 1.3) increased although
nominal yields may have decreased, as this trend in warhead development has
been accompanied by an increase in the accuracy of the delivery vehicles. When
weapon delivery accuracy is enhanced, i.e. the circular error probability (CEP)
is reduced, the weapon yield required to achieve a certain probability of destroying
a given target decreases sharply. The diagram illustrates this relationship for
probability values 0.99 and 0.9, assuming a target hardened to 10 MPa
(100 atm or 1450 psi) to be destroyed by blast from an explosion close to the
ground.

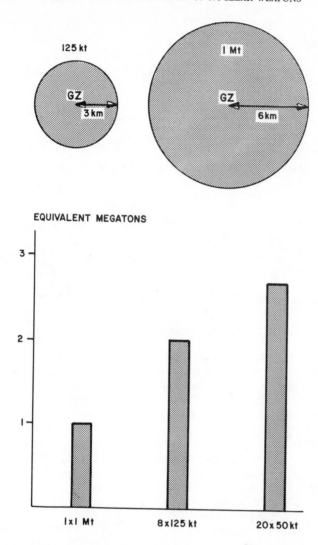

Figure 1.2. Relationship between weapon yield and area destroyed by blast. The circles illustrate how the size of the area destroyed by blast increases with weapon yield. This is accounted for by the introduction of 'equivalent megatonnage'. In the lower part of the figure are three examples of the equivalent megatonnage when the nominal yield 1 Mt. is delivered in three different ways

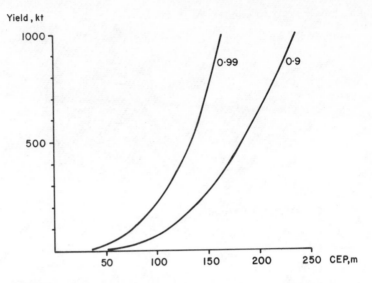

Figure 1.3. The trade-off between weapon yield and delivery accuracy

The electromagnetic pulse (EMP)

Although not a health hazard directly, the EMP can destroy radio and telephone communications over the area of a whole continent, and thus disrupt the organisation of rescue and ambulance services. Both the mechanism causing the EMP and its effect on communications are extremely complex.

A large nuclear explosion in the atmosphere disrupts radio communication both by the temporary changes produced in the ionosphere by the radiations and debris from the explosion and by creating electric fields at ground level which can damage permanently the sensitive components in transmitting and receiving equipment. The transient disturbance may last minutes or hours, but the permanent damage is much the more serious effect.

Nuclear explosions of all types produce an EMP. Those in the dense atmosphere near ground level produce very strong electric fields close to the explosion (i.e. within about 5 to 10 miles from a 1 megaton ground burst) but beyond that the damage to equipment would be small. If a nuclear weapon is exploded, however, at a height of 150 miles, the radiations emitted by the exploding core of the weapon can travel almost unimpeded through the extremely tenuous gas at that

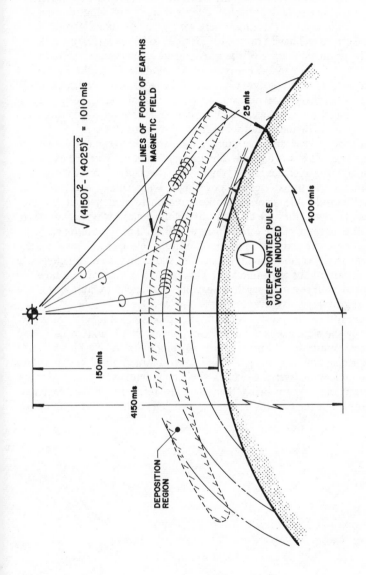

$$\sqrt{(4150)^2 - (4025)^2} = 1010\ \text{mls}$$

LINES OF FORCE OF EARTHS MAGNETIC FIELD

25 mls

4000mls

STEEP-FRONTED PULSE VOLTAGE INDUCED

150mls

4150mls

DEPOSITION REGION

Figure 1.4

height and they are stopped only when they strike the denser regions of the atmosphere and deposit their energy there. This 'deposition region' is a circular layer of the atmosphere which may be about 50 miles thick at the centre and have a mean altitude of 25 to 30 miles (Figure 1.4).

The dramatic feature of the phenomenon, however, is the radius of the deposition region. This is equal to the distance to the horizon as seen from the point of the explosion. If the latter is at an altitude of 150 miles a simple geometrical construction indicates that the horizon is more than 1000 miles away and the deposition region is a circular area of 2000 miles diameter and some 20 to 50 miles thick.

At ground level anywhere under the deposition region a potentially damaging EMP is produced. The gamma radiation from the explosion ionises air molecules as it enters the deposition region and the 'Compton electrons' ejected, covering a wide energy spectrum, can travel considerable distance in the atmosphere at that level. As they move, however, they are constrained to follow paths which rotate about the lines of force of the earth's magnetic field. The deposition region is therefore traversed by 'spokes' of orbiting electrons. These radiate energy in the radio-frequency spectrum and so induce high voltages in any aerial systems at ground level. On long power transmission lines the induced voltages may reach megavolts—sufficient to shut down the whole grid transmission system.

Very little aerial pickup is required to produce voltages which would destroy the sensitive 'solid state' components in all modern radio and telecommunications equipment, or in computers. A few high altitude explosions could therefore shut down both civilian and military communications systems over a whole continent. New equipment for military use is now being 'hardened' to resist the EMP, as far as possible, but the cost of 'hardening' existing equipment is prohibitive.

CHAPTER 2

Nuclear attack
on the United Kingdom

In this chapter we examine the form that a nuclear attack on the United Kingdom might take. The medical consequences of a nuclear attack would depend on many variables such as the number of explosions, air- or ground-burst, the time of day, the time of year and the targets selected. We review a number of possible patterns of attack on the United Kingdom from single explosions to a major nuclear exchange.

What form might a nuclear attack on the UK take?

During the course of this inquiry we discussed a number of possible forms of attack, including one in which a single nuclear weapon might be discharged against the UK by way of a warning shot. However, all but one of the experts with whom we discussed the matter said that the escalation of a conflict involving the use of nuclear weapons appeared to be inevitable. It seems extremely improbable, therefore, that an attack of the single-shot-across-the-bows type would occur, and an assessment of the medical implications of nuclear attack should be based upon more realistic contingencies.

However, it became clear that the probable scale and pattern of attack cannot be gauged with any precision. This being the case, the corollary must be that no effective planning against the consequences is possible. Nevertheless, there is some value in attempting to assess the probable order of magnitude of a nuclear attack—whether we might expect bombs with a total explosive yield of a few megatons, or of hundreds or even of thousands.

Any assessment of the probable nature and scale of a nuclear attack on the UK must take account of the strategic policies of the USA and USSR, and of the sizes and characteristics of their nuclear arsenals. Estimates of the numbers and yields of the weapons held by the nuclear

15

powers (and of the accuracies of their delivery systems) are well publicised, although there is considerable uncertainty as to the details of the various weapons systems. Targets are also classified, and we understand that developments in technology mean that target settings can be changed in a short time. Nevertheless, it is possible to specify a list of UK targets which are particularly vulnerable to attack in the context of known strategic policies.

National nuclear arsenals

Table 2.1 gives estimates of the sizes of national nuclear arsenals as at 1980, from a study commissioned by the United Nations[5]. In the case of the USA and USSR the weapons are divided into those which threaten the home territory of the opposing power, namely the central strategic weapons, the others. The UN study notes that the largest source of uncertainty in these figures concerns weapons carried by aircraft.

Table 2.1. Rough estimates of world nuclear arsenals as at 1980

Nation	'Central strategic'	Other systems	Total weapons
Number of warheads			
USA	9000–11,000	16,000–22,000	25,000–33,000
USSR	6000–7500	5000–8000	11,000–15,000
UK	NA	NA	200–1000
China	NA	NA	< 300
France	NA	NA	< 200
			37,000–50,000
Explosive yield (megatons)			
USA	3000–4000	1000–4000	4000–8000
USSR	5000–8000	2000–3000	7000–11,000
UK	NA	NA	200–1000
China	NA	NA	200–400
France	NA	NA	100
			11,000–20,000

NA = not applicable
Figures for USA and USSR rounded to nearest thousands, and for other nations to nearest hundreds. Based on open literature including *SIPRI Yearbook 1980*[10] and *The Military Balance 1979-80*[11].
Source: UN Study *Nuclear Weapons* (Frances Pinter, London, 1981)[5], Table 1, p.27.

The total world arsenal, in terms of explosive yield, is calculated here at something between 11,000 and 20,000 million tons of TNT equivalent—between three and five tons for every person on earth. Moreover, the UN report notes that calculations based on the amounts of fissile material produced by the respective countries would suggest higher total yields. Table 2.2 gives a more recent estimate of the strengths of the 'strategic' nuclear forces of the USA and the USSR.

There are important differences between 'tactical' and 'strategic' nuclear weapons. Tactical weapons are limited to a range of 15 miles or so and are intended for battlefield use. They include nuclear shells fired by artillery, bombs of the order of the explosive power of the one released over Hiroshima (now regarded as low yield), and enhanced radiation weapons, or neutron bombs. Strategic weapons include intercontinental ballistic missiles (ICBMs), submarine-launched ballistic missiles (SLBMs), free-fall bombs and air-launched missiles carried by long-range aircraft.

The picture is further complicated by the existence of 'intermediate range' or 'theatre' nuclear weapons which fall somewhere between the two earlier categories. Because 'theatre' weapons are principally deployed in Europe, they are in that context sometimes referred to as 'Eurostrategic'. The distinction between strategic and theatre weapons, either in range or explosive yield, is by no means clear, and this is a large factor contributing to the current tension over the installation of new weapons in Europe. We understand that this tension arises, in part at least, because of the geographical asymmetry between ground held by NATO and the territories of the Warsaw Pact: American 'theatre' weapons deployed by NATO in Europe can be targeted on the USSR itself, whereas equivalent Soviet weapons deployed in Warsaw Pact countries cannot reach the United States. Soviet intermediate range weapons can, of course, reach the UK and other countries in Western Europe.

It seems unlikely that a land war using tactical nuclear weapons would be conducted on British soil. Tactical weapons are designed for use in support of military operations and this is more probable, in the present political context, across the two Germanies. The nuclear threat that we may face in Britain is probably that of an attack with missiles and aircraft, employing a proportion of the USSR's strategic and 'Eurostrategic' arsenals.

The statistics given in Table 2.2 reflect a significant trend in nuclear strategy over the past two decades which has a direct bearing upon the concerns of this inquiry. Since 1965 the numbers of warheads in the US strategic arsenal have increased from about 3000 to over 9000, while the

Table 2.2. Strategic nuclear forces of the USA and the USSR in 1982

	USA			USSR		
	Number of warheads	Total yield (Mt)	Total lethality	Number of warheads	Total yield (Mt)	Total lethality
ICBMs	2152	1584	69,500	6324	3076	72,100
SLBMs	4608	181	9300	1836	792	2060
Bombers	2681	1681	—*	370	400	—*
TOTAL	9441	3446	78,800	8530	4268	74,160

*'Lethality' is a measure of the effectiveness of a nuclear weapon against a 'hard' target such as an ICBM silo. Total lethality is thus a measure of 'counterforce' capacity. Lethality depends on the yield of the warhead and, particularly, the accuracy with which it can be delivered to the target. For missiles, these accuracies can at least be estimated, and are published, for instance by the International Institute of Strategic Studies (IISS) and by the Stockholm International Peace Research Institute (SIPRI). For bombers, the concept of lethality can have no precise meaning, as it depends on factors such as air defences and crew performance.

Sources: *SIPRI Yearbook 1982*[12] (Taylor & Francis, London, 1982), Tables 7.1 and 7.2, p.269, and Appendix 7A, pp.276-280; IISS *The Military Balance 1982-83*[13], (International Institute of Strategic Studies, London, 1982), pp.112-118.

total 'lethality' (a combined measure of power and accuracy, as defined in Table 2.2) has increased from about 3000 to nearly 80,000. An even more striking trend is apparent for the USSR, where the number of warheads has risen from about 700 to more than 8000 over the same period. Yet the lethality of the Russian arsenal has increased from barely 300 in 1965[6] to well over 70,000 in 1982.

There has clearly been a strong move away from (relatively) few weapons of high yield but low accuracy, suitable for threatening large targets such as cities, towards much larger numbers of weapons of rather lower yield but very much greater accuracy, designed for attacking strategic military targets. Current developments of new weapons systems of even greater accuracy accentuate this trend. These technological developments in weapons with increasing counterforce capability, as distinct from simple deterrence, have been accompanied by corresponding changes in strategic policies.

The inference now is that it is much more likely that an initial nuclear attack on the UK would be primarily, perhaps even exclusively, of the 'counterforce' type—directed against military targets rather than cities as such. This would mean the use of large numbers of warheads with yields of a megaton or less against targets dispersed all over the UK (many of them in or close to densely populated areas) rather than fewer multi-megaton warheads directed at major cities. A significant proportion of the detonations in such an attack would be of the 'ground-burst' type defined in the previous section. The effectiveness of a counterforce attack would depend upon there being little or no warning, which means that casualties of the kind discussed in Chapter 3 would tend to be higher than if there were a warning period of several days or even weeks.

Table 2.3 gives details of Soviet nuclear weapons in the 'strategic' category as at mid-1982 and shows that their total explosive power amounts to over 4000 million tons of TNT equivalent. Several of these missile types carry more than one warhead—they have 'multiple re-entry vehicles' (MRVs). In some cases these can be separately targeted —they are 'multiple independently targetable re-entry vehicles' (MIRVs).

Table 2.4 gives figures for Soviet 'primary Eurostrategic', or longer-range, 'theatre' nuclear weapons known to exist in 1982. These missiles carry warheads with a total yield of nearly 500 megatons. It is more

Table 2.3. Soviet strategic nuclear weapons as at mid-1982

Vehicle	Number deployed	Number of warheads	Total yield (Mt)
ICBMs:			
SS11/2	230	230	230
SS11/3	290	870	174
SS13	60	60	60
SS17	150	600	300
SS18	308	2464	1232
SS19	360	2160	1080
SLBMs:			
SSN5	18	18	18
SSN6/2	102	102	102
SSN6/3	272	544	109
SSN8	290	290	290
SSNX17	12	12	12
SSN18	256	768	154
Aircraft:			
Mya 4	56	112	112
Tu 95	100	300	300
Total			4173

Source: *SIPRI Yearbook 1982* [12], Appendix 7A, pp.276–280; Table 7.1, p.269.

Table 2.4. Primary Soviet longer-range ('Eurostrategic') nuclear weapons, 1982

Vehicle	Number deployed	Number of warheads	Total yield (Mt)
IRBMs:*			
SS4	275	275	275
SS5	16	16	16
SS20	315	945	142
SLBMs:			
SSN5	57	57	57
			490
Aircraft:†			
Tu 16	310	310	310
Tu 22	125	125	125
Tu 22M	100	100	100
			535
TOTAL			1025

Sources: IISS *The Military Balance 1982-83* [13], pp.112-118; *SIPRI Yearbook 1982* [12], pp.3-50.
*According to the SIPRI, about two-thirds of the IRBMs are deployed in the European theatre and about three-quarters of the medium-range aircraft.
†In line with IISS and SIPRI practice, naval air force bombers are not included in the table, nor are shorter-range nuclear-capable 'strike aircraft'.

difficult to estimate the numbers and total yield of warheads carried by aircraft. Estimates are usually based upon known payloads (weapon loads) of the aircraft concerned, but there can be big discrepancies according to whether the criterion used is the 'operational load' or the 'maximum load'. Also, it is not known for certain how many aircraft are actually deployed on these duties, nor what proportion of them are assigned to the European theatre. If the weapons carried by the aircraft in Table 2.4 are included, the total yield of Soviet 'primary Eurostrategic' warheads probably exceeds 1000 megatons.

Estimates of the possible scale of an attack

To calculate the maximum weight of an attack on Britain, it is necessary to determine what proportion of Russian strategic weapons might be assigned to Western Europe, and then divide these, along with the

'Eurostrategic' weapons, between the countries of Europe. However, there are massive imponderables, such as whether or not all the weapons in the Soviet arsenal would be used, and how many of the weapons actually launched might succeed in reaching their target.

Despite these uncertainties, some independent observers have made theoretical calculations in order to arrive at plausible levels of attack as a basis for discussion. Goodwin (1981)[7], for instance, assumes that none of the Russian strategic ICBM or long-range bomber forces would be used in Europe, and that no tactical weapons would be used against Britain. Excluding tactical nuclear weapons leaves the missiles and aircraft listed in Table 2.3. Working from estimates published in *The Military Balance 1980–1981*[8], Goodwin obtains a total of close on 2000 warheads which might be available for use against Western Europe. Of these, he suggests some 800 might reach their targets, making allowance for aircraft being shot down and missile failures.

Distributing these weapons between the NATO countries on the basis of their respective populations, Goodwin expects 140 warheads to be used against Britain. The explosive power of these warheads would be 150 kilotons for the SS20s, 1 megaton for the SS4s and SS5s, and possibly more powerful weapons carried by the bombers. A figure for total yield of 100–150 megatons seems to be the conclusion of this analysis. A possible weakness of this formula is the argument that Britain, being a nuclear power in its own right, as well as accommodating many important United States bases, could well attract more than its fair share of weapons on a strict per capita reckoning.

Clarke (1982)[9] takes a different approach. He starts from an assessment of likely targets in Britain (based on a reading of Soviet military doctrine) and goes on to assign to each of these one or more weapons with specified yields. On this basis he calculates the expenditure of 127 megatons on military and industrial targets, plus another 40 megatons on otherwise untargeted cities, giving a total weight of 167 megatons.

A recent study of global nuclear war sponsored by the Royal Swedish Academy of Sciences journal *Ambio*[14] depicts a scenario in which roughly half the world's total projected 1985 arsenal of strategic and tactical weapons is detonated—some 15,000 warheads, totalling 5750 megatons. The reason that this admittedly catastrophic scenario features only half the world arsenal is that the authors found it impossible to identify 'reasonable' targets for any more weapons. This is a scenario which features military, industrial/economic and population targets. Cities in Western Europe are allocated explosive yields of one megaton per 100,000 to one million population; three megatons for a population of between one and three million; and ten megatons for a city of upwards of three million people. According to this formula, cities in the UK could anticipate receiving about 80 megatons, leaving aside all further military and industrial targeting.

Openshaw and Steadman (1983a)[15] quote another study which takes actual Soviet 'Eurostrategic' and strategic weapons and assigns them principally to military targets, according to priorities mentioned in Soviet strategic literature. A few industrial targets are also included, but no cities are targeted as such. The number of warheads used (340) is greater than in the other studies so far cited with the inclusion of some 44 SS20s each with three MIRVed warheads together with seven SS19s, each with six MIRVed warheads. Most of the other warheads used are in 1 Mt yield. However, the total megatonnage, (222 Mt) is comparable with other assessments including a figure which recurs in Home Office literature. The result is a relatively low average yield per weapon (0.65 Mt).

Recently, for purposes of home defence training, the Home Office seems to have been working on the assumption of an attack around the 200-megaton mark. In the introduction to its *Training Manual for Scientific Advisers* (1977)[16], the Home Office predicts:

If the Warsaw Pact Nations constitute the enemy—and this is only one possible assumption—and if the enemy directs the bulk of his medium-range and intermediate-range weapons against targets in Western Europe behind the battle-front, then Western Europe would receive about 1000 megatons. Perhaps the UK could expect about one-fifth of this, say 200 Mt.

The same figure is reiterated in another Home Office publication, *Domestic Nuclear Shelters: Technical Guidance* (1981)[17], while Home Office Scientific Advisory Branch computer studies have evaluated the effects of attack with yields of 193 and 181 megatons. Meanwhile, the September 1980 Home Defence exercise code-named 'Square Leg' postulated an attack with 125 weapons, with a combined yield of approximately 200 megatons.

Commenting on these Home Office and 'Square Leg' 200 megaton estimates, Rogers, in Dando and Newman, eds, (1982)[19], insisted that 'this seems an extremely low figure and one which we find very difficult to take seriously'. As he says, it represents 'less than 3 per cent of Soviet medium- and long-range warhead systems and less than 5 per cent of megatonnage, and this for a country with a unique concentration of targets'.

In evidence to the Working Party on these issues the Ministry of

Defence could offer no quantitative estimates. The question was asked:

Do you think . . . that an attack would be balanced evenly across the NATO countries? That is something people point out: there are sixteen countries all facing Russia. Would you expect the same number of missiles dropped on to each of them, or would one country, like the UK, expect a predominantly heavier attack?

The spokesman for the Ministry replied that:

. . . in regard to the pattern of attack on NATO countries I think this is, quite frankly, impossible to predict, and I know of no precise prediction in the Ministry of Defence. I think it is fairly clear as to why there could not possibly be one. On the other hand, I think it is fairly safe to say that we cannot expect any degree of immunity being provided to one country or another within the Alliance . . . . So much depends on the particular crisis scenario, but the United Kingdom is a very important reinforcement base, in terms of our own forces reinforcing mainland Europe and in terms of enabling the United States, in many circumstances, to reinforce mainland Europe.

He agreed that the fact of the UK being used as a staging post for US forces in war would provide a reason for this country being a specially important target.

That is one reason, among others. There are others in terms of our own military capabilities, in terms of our own maritime defence over the North Sea and the Channel approaches. All of these factors would make us a potent threat to the Soviets in the event of a war, and, given that, if it became necessary to their objectives in the event of a conflict, then they would have to consider a nuclear attack.

We asked the Home Office what scale of attack was envisaged for the purposes of home defence plans and whether for example the 'Square Leg' exercise could be taken as a guide to Home Office thinking. The Home Office spokesman replied:

Taking as a starting point the 'Square Leg' scenario, it was a scenario devised for no purpose and on no basis other than to give training opportunities to people who were being exercised. It in no way reflects our assessment of the possible scale of attack the Soviet Union might launch against this country if a war in Europe developed into a nuclear war. It has of course been given an importance and significance quite different from that. Nuclear disarmament and peace movements have said that this is an accurate prediction by the Government of the scale of attack which they expect to be launched against this country. It could not be because we do not know.

If their [the Soviet Union's] objective was . . . to achieve certain aims such as the neutralisation of West Germany or to improve their political position in Western Europe, then their attack on this country would almost certainly be confined to [that] attack necessary to limit the flow of British and American reinforcements to the mainland of Europe. In that case they would attack military targets or airfields and centres of communication and so on which were of military value. If their objective was to remove this country from future political and economic reckoning in Europe, they might attack centres of industry and of commerce and indeed, even population . . . I am not sure what scale of attack they would consider it necessary to launch if this was their aim. A 'Square Leg' attack of what was about 200 megatons on about 80 targets would certainly cause tremendous disruption a long time in the future, and they would have it within their power to launch much larger attacks — perhaps 1000 or 2000 megatons.

Asked to give a figure for the *maximum* conceivable level of attack on Britain, another Home Office representative mentioned 3000 megatons as the heaviest bombardment studied using the Scientific Advisory Branch's computer model. The results of this analysis are reported briefly in Butler (1981)[18]. Butler, however, regards an attack of this magnitude as 'clearly not defensible on military grounds'. He implies that it was investigated purely as a theoretical exercise.

Ground-launched cruise missiles as targets

The question arises as to whether the proposed siting of ground-launched cruise missiles in the UK during 1983 (at Greenham Common near Newbury, and at Molesworth near Huntingdon) might influence the level of attack. Ground launched cruise missiles (GLCMs), carried on mobile launchers, are intended to be moved a distance of anything up to 100 miles from their bases in preparation for use. Not surprisingly, therefore, it has been argued that an aggressor might bombard the entire area of their possible deployment, in order to ensure the destruction of these missiles.

In 1981, Geoffrey Pattie, Secretary of State for Defence (Air Force), stated in a written reply to a parliamentary question on this point, that 'more than 1000 megatons would be needed to destroy the ground-launched cruise missiles once they were dispersed'. Apparently this figure is obtained by a theoretical calculation of the total yield of bombs needed to carpet the entire deployment area at a specified blast damage level.

Dr Frank Barnaby gave evidence to the working party on this whole question of the possible weight of attack. He was asked his opinion of the realism of the 'Square Leg' scenario. He also took into account the possible consequences of the deployment of cruise missiles. He proposed that:

A good basic rule of thumb would be five tons per head of population. So for the British population this would mean 300 megatons on that basis. But because England has so many bases and is so strategically important, one would have to double that realistically, so 600 megatons would be the figure I would go for, which is mid-way between the 'Square Leg' 200 and the figure of 3000 which has been mentioned officially. I think 3000 is probably too much. As to the deployment of the cruise missiles here, possibly one could argue for more than 600 megatons, but if one said 600 megatons that would be a figure that could not seriously be criticised.

The majority of the opinion given to the Working Party inclined to the view that an attack might amount to 150 or 200 megatons; with a total of three or four times this magnitude if cruise missiles were to be deployed in the United Kingdom.

'Limited' attacks

The figures in Table 2.5 represent different estimates of a credible level of nuclear attack on Britain. It is nevertheless also valuable to examine the possibility of lower levels of bombardment, for instance, an attack restricted to a few military objectives, accurately targeted, with cities and industry supposedly spared, or an attack launched against a single city, say, or with a single weapon, in some form of nuclear blackmail or demonstration of intent or even by accident. The implications of the single-shot scenario are vastly different from those of all-out nuclear war.

The various scenarios produce entirely different medical effects. The implications for the role and effectiveness of Home Defence are also completely different. With a single bomb, or even possibly an attack limited to one part of the country, resources could be mobilised to help the survivors from the 'outside'. In a comprehensive attack on the country as a whole, there would be no 'outside'.

Table 2.5. Estimated level of attack on the UK by the USSR

Author	Warheads	Targets	Total megatons
Goodwin (1981)[7]	140	114	
Clarke (1982)[9]	188		167
Ambio (1982) (cities only)[14]			80
Openshaw and Steadman (1983)[20]	340		222
Home Office (1977, 1981)[16,17]		80	200
'Square Leg' exercise 1980	125	100	200
Home Office (Butler, 1982)[18]	84		181
Home Office	179		193
Home Office (hypothetical maximum on computer model)			3000
Barnaby (BMA evidence, assumes deployment of GLCMs)			600

The credibility of 'limited' nuclear war

The Working Party was told that NATO policy in Europe is constructed on the theory of 'flexible response', in which the scale and nature of attack can be matched and so, in theory, deterred at each of a graduated series of levels: tactical weapons met with tactical weapons, theatre or intermediate range missiles met with their equivalent, an attack on NATO military bases countered by an attack on comparable Soviet bases, and so on. The realism or feasibility of setting such notional limits of self-restraint on the conduct of warfare have been repeatedly cast into doubt over the last twenty years both by military commanders and strategic theorists.

Professor Zuckerman, former Chief Scientific Adviser to the Ministry of Defence, reviews the opinions of a number of commentators in his book *Nuclear Illusion and Reality* (1982)[21]. He points out that no less than five out of seven holders of the post of Chief of Defence Staff in Britain since 1957 have declared themselves sceptical about the whole concept of limited nuclear warfare. As long ago as 1960, Capt Basil Liddell Hart argued that if tactical nuclear weapons were used on the battlefield, the result would very likely be an escalation 'precipitating an illimitable and suicidal H-bomb devastation of countries and cities'.

The most widely known statement is that of the late Lord Mountbatten, who in 1979 said that the belief that nuclear weapons 'could be used in warfare without triggering an all-out nuclear exchange leading to the final holocaust . . . is more and more incredible. I cannot accept the reasons for the belief that any class of nuclear weapons can be categorised in terms of their tactical or strategic purposes. In all sincerity, as a military man I can see no use for any nuclear weapons which would not end in escalation, with consequences that no one can conceive.'

In 1962 Helmut Schmidt, former Chancellor of West Germany, wrote: 'Defence against a non-nuclear aggression in Europe with the aid of tactical nuclear weapons, even in the unlikely event of both sides keeping within bounds and avoiding the upward acceleration of weapons, would most probably mean the extensive destruction of Europe and, at all events, of Germany.'

Zuckerman says that simulations and war games relating to tactical nuclear war in Europe overwhelmingly indicate that the results would be catastrophic and in all likelihood uncontrollable. He quotes the former US Assistant Secretary of Defence Alan Enthoven to the effect that: 'Tactical nuclear weapons cannot defend Europe; they can only destroy it . . . . Because of the vulnerability of key forces, the big advantages to striking first, and the location near cities of many airfields, transportation links, command posts and the like, the likelihood of escalation would be very high . . . there is no such thing as a two-sided tactical nuclear war in the sense of sustained purposive military operations . . . nobody knows how to fight a tactical nuclear war. Twenty years of effort by many military experts have failed to produce a believable doctrine for tactical nuclear warfare.'

On the question of whether the Soviet Union subscribes to any concept of graduated nuclear war, Zuckerman argues that this is not the case. Suggestions sometimes made that the Russians believe in the possibility of fighting and 'winning' a nuclear war are based he feels on a misreading of Soviet military writings and in particular Marshal Sokolovski's influential *Military Strategy*[22]. Direct questioning by Zuckerman of General Mikhail Milshtein on this point produced the answer that 'The men at the top of the USSR understand the incredible dangers just as much as your leaders do. No one can win with nuclear weapons.' It seems that Soviet military doctrine, so far from envisaging restraint once the nuclear threshold is crossed, on the contrary according to SIPRI[12] 'emphasises initiative, surprise, deep strikes and massive use.'

We discussed these conflicting opinions with many of the experts and government spokesman who met the members of the Working Party.

In oral evidence to the Working Party, the Ministry of Defence appears to argue the rationale of 'flexible response':

The whole business of the Ministry of Defence in the first place is deterrence, and it is only if deterrence fails that we expect to have to resort to the other aspect of NATO policy, which is defence. Even there it would always be aimed at restoring the deterrent, hopefully before it came to a nuclear war; and even if the worst happens, and one side or the other uses nuclear weapons, we would still hope to be able to restore deterrence before there is more nuclear war. We do not necessarily regard it as the most likely scenario that there would have to be all-out nuclear war.

Amplifying this point, another spokesman for the Ministry said:

We have no intention of fighting, obviously, any sort of nuclear war, limited or otherwise, but we recognise that once it started there are enormous dangers of it escalating into strategic exchange. But as [we have] said, if it did start, that is not necessarily the end of the road. It would still be NATO's policy to try and stop the war as soon as possible.

The Home Office spokesman, however, clearly thought that a nuclear exchange could be contained at some limited level.

On the question of escalation, people like Carver and Mountbatten are reported to have said that once an exchange of nuclear weapons began, even on the battlefield, it would almost inevitably escalate to an all-out strategic nuclear exchange. As far as I know they produced no logical basis for that assumption. It seems equally likely that once an exchange of battlefield weapons had begun in Europe, or even an exchange of [theatre] weapons directed against the UK or Eastern Europe, at that point the main antagonists could well draw back appalled at the possible consequences of what might happen.

The Home Office representative elaborated on the possibility of the Soviet Union launching an airborne attack on the UK with conventional bombs (or possibly chemical weapons) in the first place, and, finding that unsuccessful, progressing to the use of nuclear weapons, perhaps of relatively low yield. The representative went on to describe the possibility of a limited nuclear attack, intended to prevent the reinforcement from Britain of NATO forces in Europe. The attack would be directed predominantly at east coast ports and airfields in East Anglia. Such an attack might involve some 50 to 100 bombs, with yields perhaps in the kiloton range.

A spokesman for the Arms Control and Disarmament Research Unit of the Foreign and Commonwealth Office (FCO), on the other hand, pointed out the important difference between nuclear explosions over Soviet satellite countries and over the Soviet homeland. He was equivocal about the possibility of a limited nuclear war in Europe on the grounds that: '. . . the Soviet Union has said that any US missile falling on Soviet territory would be treated as coming from the United States and would draw a reaction in response against the United States' territory.'

He did not imagine that a nuclear war, once initiated at some low level, would necessarily be uncontrollable. The use of tactical weapons against Soviet formations in Germany, for example, would not automatically result in retaliation by Russia elsewhere than in Germany. As for dropping bombs on Russian territory itself:

FCO   'But when you are talking about dropping [nuclear weapons] on Russian homeland, remember the point we have made categorically that no NATO weapons will ever be used in Europe except in response to an attack, so the idea of delivering a nuclear weapon against the Soviet Union from Europe is ruled out.'

BMA   'Offensive, yes. What I am trying to clear up is, if by mistake or on purpose or in some way hostilities reach a certain threshold where nuclear weapons have been used, then escalation and all-out exchange is, in your view, not at all impossible?"

FCO   'Once you start on the ladder of escalation, then it is a very slippery slope.'

BMA   'Is it an escalating slope?'

FCO   'No: one can visualise a stage in which both parties will pause and scratch their heads and say "What are we doing?" '

In contrast, Frank Barnaby's opinion is that 'a limited nuclear war is simply not on'. He supports this view, as others have done, with the argument that the technological characteristics of new weapons systems make the control of any escalation much more problematic. The accuracy of these weapons creates pressure for their immediate use, even for their 'launch on warning' of an incoming attack, since otherwise there is a danger they may be destroyed in place before they can be fired in return. 'The crucial thing at the moment — the thing that makes the 1980s unique — is the new weapons . . . . The crucial point about these new ones [MX, the Cruise missile, new tactical weapons] is that they are nuclear-war-fighting, and a nuclear-war-fighting strategy requires a rather rapid escalation. So we are moving into a period of more rapid escalation. The sort of scenario that we are thinking of is a war which begins with a tactical nuclear war in Europe but quite rapidly escalates to a strategic nuclear exchange which itself rapidly escalates so that most of the arsenals would be used in a fairly short time.'

We cannot escape the conclusion that the use of nuclear weapons at any level would probably escalate into a major strategic conflict in which the United Kingdom would be heavily involved. In such a case we might expect to suffer nuclear explosions over the UK roughly in accordance with the weapons and yields set out in Tables 2.3 and 2.4. The medical effects of such an attack, both in relation to a single explosion and to the combined effects of a series of explosions, are discussed in Chapters 3 and 4.

CHAPTER 3

Mortality and morbidity
consequent upon a nuclear attack

Part A of this chapter deals with the medical effects of a nuclear explosion up to 14–21 days after an attack. Details are given of the types of injury that might be expected, and their causes.

Abstracts from the British Medical Journal are quoted in Annex 3 to illustrate standards and methods of medical care that have been applied to the treatment of victims of one recent civil disaster and one recent high-explosive bomb attack in this country. These are contrasted with predictions for the number of deaths and injuries following the detonation of nuclear weapons over the United Kingdom.

Estimations for the number of casualties resulting from different types of attack are examined in Part B. There are discrepancies between the projections for blast, heat and radiation produced by the Scientific Advisory Branch of the Home Office and by the organisation Scientists Against Nuclear Arms.

Part A   Injuries following a nuclear explosion

The three main effects of a nuclear explosion which kill and injure people are blast, heat and ionising radiation. For air-bursts in the megaton range and for city targets it is blast and heat that kill or injure the largest number of people. In the case of a ground-burst many more casualties may result from radiation days or weeks after the explosion. These later casualties may eventually exceed those from all other causes. This is because fall-out can cover much larger areas than those devastated by blast or fire.

The United Nations Comprehensive Study on Nuclear Weapons describes the effects on people who are in the vicinity of a nuclear explosion as follows:

When a nuclear weapon is exploded above ground, the first noticeable effect is a blinding flash of intense white light, strong enough to temporarily blind or at least dazzle observers many kilometres distant from the explosion. The general impression is that the whole sky is brilliantly illuminated. The light is emitted from the surface of the 'fireball', a roughly spherical mass of very hot air and weapon residues, which develops quickly around the exploding weapon and continues to grow until it reaches a maximum radius which depends on the yield. For a weapon with a yield of 10 to 20 kt, i.e. that of the Hiroshima and Nagasaki bombs, the maximum radius is approximately 200 m. and its development takes about one second. During that time, and for some time after, the fireball emits thermal radiation both as light and — mainly — heat. Finally, the thermal radiation dies away as the fireball is cooled and transformed into the mushroom-shaped explosion cloud. By then, about one third of the explosive energy has been released as heat. Within and close to the fireball, everything will evaporate or melt. At some distance from the explosion the two most important effects of thermal radiation will be to cause burns ('flash burns') on exposed skin and to ignite fires. Second-degree burns to unprotected skin may occur 3 km. from the explosion, and at 2 km. third-degree burns will be frequent. (Second-degree burns cause pain and blisters. Third-degree burns, where parts of the skin are destroyed, cause disfiguring scars called cheloids.) At less than 2 km., thermal radiation can be expected to kill most people directly exposed to it. Materials that are easily ignited, such as thin fabrics, paper or dry leaves, may catch fire at more than 2 km. from ground-zero. This may cause numerous fires, which under some conditions may form a huge fire storm enveloping much of the target area and adding numerous further casualties. That was the case in Hiroshima, although it is considered less likely in modern cities.

Often the most important effect of a nuclear explosion is the blast wave, which is similar to that of a chemical explosion but differs quantitatively owing to the much larger amount of energy involved. The air blast carries about half the explosive energy (see Figure 1.1) and travels much slower than the various forms of radiation, but — for the yield chosen here — in about one and a half seconds it reaches a 1 km. circle around ground-zero and in 5 or 6 seconds it has expanded to 3 km. The arrival of the blast wave is experienced as a sudden and shattering blow, immediately followed by a hurricane-force wind directed outwards from the explosion. Out to perhaps 1.5 km. from ground-zero, where the maximum wind speed will be about 90 m./sec. (three times 'full gale' by the meteorological definition), the blast wind may uproot trees, blow down telephone and utility poles and overturn even heavy (civilian) vehicles. Virtually all buildings will be utterly demolished. Persons standing in the open will be swept up by the wind and carried with it along the surface of the ground, hitting other objects and being hit by loose, flying debris which acts as projectiles, killing or injuring people. Out to a distance of at least 2 m. most buildings will be crushed by the compressional load as they are engulfed by the blast overpressure and the wind drag. People inside may be crushed under the weight of the falling buildings, hurt by the flying debris of broken windows, furniture, etc, or even suffocated by the dense dust of crushed brick and mortar. Especially in houses that are partially damaged, fires may start from overturned stoves and fires, broken gas lines, etc, causing further casualties among the population. A very rough estimate is that within the 1.5 km.-circle, the blast will kill — by various mechanisms — virtually everybody in the open or in ordinary buildings. All the primary blast destruction has taken place during a few seconds.

Radiation

As the bomb explodes, intense ionising radiation consisting primarily of neutrons and gamma rays is emitted. Up to a mile and a half away unprotected victims receive a lethal dose, but those this close to the explosion would be killed by blast and heat.

Radiation sickness

The most important longer-term effect of ground or near-surface bursts is fall-out. Over a period of a few hours after detonation, unprotected people as far as 80 to 160 kilometres downwind of the explosion may receive a lethal dose of radiation from fall-out. Although high doses of radiation have been extensively studied in experimental animals (and there is detailed evidence of the effects of fairly low doses of radiation in humans), knowledge of the effects of high doses on the human body in circumstances similar to those of a nuclear war is based on small numbers of incidents in which individuals have been accidentally exposed to radiation. In Japan large numbers of people were exposed to a range of doses of radiation but the observations made were incomplete and were complicated by the effects of combined injuries. The experience of radiation in medical treatment, for example in the treatment of cancer and in bone marrow transplantation, does not contribute a great deal to the calculation of the likely mortality from radiation exposure in nuclear war.

At comparatively low whole-body doses of radiation (under about 1 Gy), anorexia, nausea and vomiting are common but no deaths are likely in a physically fit population. Above this dose bone marrow damage occurs. Without treatment there is considerable uncertainty about the lethal dose for 50 per cent mortality (LD 50) in humans. However, it is thought to be around 4–4½ Gy. Above 6 Gy survival is unlikely.

The effects of radiation on bone marrow have been well described by Andrews in 'Medical Management of Accidental Total Body Irradiation'[23].

Decrease in lymphocytes occurs promptly, most of it taking place within 24 hours after exposure. The level of this early lymphopoenia is one of the best indicators as to severity of radiation injury. The level of neutrophil granulocytes shows a very early rise usually limited to the first 48 hours or less but the degree of elevation has not been correlated with the extent of injury. In the dose range producing the haematopoietic syndrome, after the early rise, granulocyte numbers fall to fairly low levels at about day 10 and there is a transient abortive rise at about day 15, perhaps due to mitosis of a genetically damaged cell population which cannot continue to reproduce. (The absence of an abortive rise is an unfavourable sign.) There is then a steady fall in granulocyte count beginning at about day 30 after exposure if the patient survives, which is followed by a spontaneous recovery beginning in the fifth week. The platelets may show a rise in the first two or three days after exposure, then a gradually accelerating decrease with the nadir also reached at about day 30. During the recovery the platelets usually rise to well above normal levels.

Several factors are likely to affect the LD 50. Dose rate is certainly important and breaking a given dose up into units increases the total dose which can be tolerated. If a dose of radiation is received over a longer period the LD 50 will be raised. Radiation of only part of the body would also affect the LD 50, as shielding part of the marrow increases the probability of survival. At the extremes of life sensitivity to radiation is increased. In the case of children, a larger dose of radiation would be received by the bone marrow for a given external dose than in adults.

Diarrhoea and other gastro-intestinal symptoms were common effects of radiation in Hiroshima and Nagasaki and decreased with the distance from ground zero. Bloody diarrhoea was noted in about 10 per cent of those within one kilometre of ground zero at the time of attack and in one per cent beyond five kilometres. However, studies of radiation given to facilitate bone marrow grafts suggest that quite high doses of radiation can be tolerated without producing gastro-intestinal symptoms. It is generally thought that severe gastro-intestinal symptoms result from doses of radiation in the range from 5–20 Gy. The effects are due to inhibition of mitosis of the cells in intestinal crypts. This causes electrolyte loss and bacterial invasion. Death is likely to result from a combination of fluid loss and secondary infection.

Very high doses of radiation above 20 Gy produce the 'neurovascular syndrome' in which there may be a short interval of mental alertness before victims become comatose and die. At very high dose ranges of above 70 Gy the period of mental alertness before coma may be very short.

There are other clinically significant short-term effects of radiation. High doses may be received if skin is contaminated by beta emitting particles in fall-out, and radiation erythema may appear after a dose of about 3 Gy to the skin. The dose at which erythema starts to appear is somewhat lower for neutron exposure. At doses above 10 Gy, scaling, blistering and ulcerative changes may all occur and if the patient survives long enough there may be keloid formation. 'Beta burns' were seen amongst some of the Marshall islanders exposed to radiation after the 1954 Bravo test explosion. Hair-loss may occur after a dose to the scalp of 3 Gy or more. Recovery takes place in the months following exposure unless the hair follicles have been exposed to high doses.

Fertility is likely to be impaired following radiation exposure. The testes are radio-sensitive. A dose as low as 0.1 Gy can depress sperm production for up to a year and 2.5 Gy will produce sterility for three years or longer. The ovary is more radio-resistant but doses of 1-2 Gy will cause temporary sterility.

At Hiroshima and Nagasaki it was noted that children exposed to radiation *in utero* tended to be smaller than average. Amongst 169 children exposed *in utero* at Hiroshima there were 33 with microcephaly (defined as two or more standard deviations below normal). About half of these were mentally retarded. Another survey[24] of 487 persons exposed *in utero* to radiation at Hiroshima and Nagasaki and 1,010 children (used as a control group) whose mothers were not exposed showed that the frequency of microcephaly increased with radiation dosage. Thirty-seven mothers who had received over 0.5 Gy within the eighteenth week of gestation bore 16 children with microcephaly. Amongst 13 children whose mothers had been exposed to over 1.5 Gy five were microcephalic and mentally retarded. In Hiroshima the minimum dose producing microcephaly was 0.1-0.19 Gy but no mentally regarded microcephalic children were observed under 1.5 Gy in Nagasaki. Microcephaly was frequently accompanied by mental retardation at paternal doses of more than 1.5 Gy in both cities. The difference between the two cities may be because the atomic bomb dropped on Hiroshima emitted more neutron radiation than the weapon used at Nagasaki.

In a nuclear war it is likely that many victims will suffer from the combined effects of radiation, burns and blast and consequently injuries which may be relatively minor under normal circumstances could be fatal when combined with others of similar severity, particularly in the absence of adequate treatment and basic sanitation.

The psychological effects

During the post attack phase, those who survived the immediate effects of nuclear bombardment would be under immense stress. The psychological effects of such an attack (and their influence on the ability of survivors to cope with bereavement, physical suffering, devastated environment and associated problems) are difficult to predict with certainty. However, the experiences of Hiroshima and Nagasaki suggest that many people would be incapable of organised activity. For instance, Hachiya, a Japanese physician at Hiroshima[27], wrote:

Parents, half-crazy with grief, search for their children. Husbands look for their wives, and children for their parents. One poor woman, insane with anxiety walked aimlessly here and there through the hospital calling her child's name. What a weak fragile thing man is before the forces of destruction. After the flash the entire population had been reduced to a common level of physical and mental weakness. Those who were able walked silently towards suburbs and distant hills, their spirits broken, their initiative gone. When asked whence they had come, they pointed to the City and said 'That way', and when asked where they were going they pointed away from the city and said, 'This way'. They were so broken and confused that they moved and behaved like automatons.

It has been pointed out that social disorganisation is more marked when there is little warning of disaster and when the destruction is greater and less clearly understood. The psychological consequences of fall-out could be extremely important. It has been shown in previous studies of disasters that threats or dangers which cannot be reliably perceived by the senses can cause considerable psychological disturbance. For example, a mass poisoning by boot-leg whisky in Georgia, USA, led to large numbers of people attending casualty departments. When tested, about 40 per cent were unaffected by lethal alcohol and some of these confessed that they did not know whether or not they were affected but wanted to be checked. After a nuclear attack, many people might wish to be reassured that they had not been exposed to appreciable levels of radiation. This could add to the already chaotic situation surrounding hospitals and treatment centres, if these were still available.

For those in shelters there would be the great strain of not knowing the whereabouts or safety of friends and relatives. There would be the temptation to emerge prematurely from cover to look for them. It would not be clear in many instances whether those with nausea, vomiting and diarrhoea were merely suffering from intercurrent infection resulting in gastro-enteritis or whether they were victims of potentially fatal radiation sickness. This uncertainty would add appreciably to their stress.

It has been suggested from the study of other disasters that perhaps 12 to 25 per cent of victims would remain relatively calm during a disaster, whereas about 75 per cent would be temporarily stunned and bewildered. This bewildered state might persist long after the disaster, causing apathy, aimlessness and depression. A small proportion of people might display inappropriate responses to the trauma including confusion, severe anxiety, hysterical screaming or aggression. Although there are large individual variations in response to severe stress it is likely that a nuclear attack would prove such a powerful stimulus that it would influence the behaviour of even the most robust survivor.

Lifton and Olsen[28], who studied the survivors of the Buffalo Creek flood disaster in West Virginia in 1972, showed that the complete destruction of the social fabric of that community led to psychological impairment in all survivors studied two years after the flood. At this time there was still evidence of despair, apathy and depression and a constrictive living pattern among survivors. Also, they described frequent memory lapses and confusion about the details of events since the disaster. In many cases there was impairment of interpersonal relationships and many survivors remained very suspicious of all forms of help. Some people were able to focus anger on the mining company responsible for the burst dam, but others felt the necessity to project their anger onto individuals. Much of the Buffalo Creek survivors' anger and bitterness appeared to be due to their inability to come to terms with the apparent lack of meaning of a disaster which had seemed to be preventable. There was a loss of any sense of moral rectitude and it appeared to them that the mining company had gone unpunished.

The incidence of long-term psychological disability following major disasters varies. For instance, follow-up studies[39] of survivors of Cyclone Tracy in Darwin, Australia, showed that 41 per cent of those people involved had psychological disfunctioning ten weeks after the cyclone (a decrease from 58 per cent initially). By 14 months psychological disfunctioning had returned to the general population control level of 22 per cent. On the other hand, follow-up of 300 survivors of World War II prison and concentration camps showed that all of them had disabling psychiatric symptoms many years afterwards. It is quite likely that similar reactions would follow a nuclear war. In fact the psychological effects of attack might well increase the demand for such medical services as did manage to survive.

Treatment following a nuclear war

During World War II considerable experience was obtained in all aspects of the management of air raid and military casualties. In major cities the number of casualties was high, but the rescue teams, ambulance services and hospitals were able to deal with the problems adequately and efficiency increased with experience. The emphasis on getting casualties to hospital with the minimum of delay was found to be life-saving. In civilian practice, treatment at the site of the incident was found to be impracticable in the conditions prevailing during air-raids.

In hospital, reception and assessment of the seriously injured for priority treatment (triage) was the most important initial process in medical management. It became common experience that if a patient could be admitted to hospital alive the prospects of survival were good. These lessons have proved to be true in civil disasters and in bomb attacks in the UK in the 1970s and 1980s. Three papers from the British Medical Journal are set out in Annex 3. Together, they illustrate the methods and standards of treatment that are currently considered to be desirable for victims of blast and other traumatic injuries. This is the response that doctors and nurses strive to give through the National Health Service to the whole range of injuries, serious and minor in extent, that may follow the detonation of a high explosive bomb or some other major disaster. The hospital beds allocated for acute care in England and Wales are listed by Region in Table 3.1.

Table 3.1   Available acute beds by region (1978)

1.	Northern	9564
2.	Yorkshire	11,034
3.	Trent	9434
4.	East Anglia	4679
5.	North West Thames	10,333
6.	North East Thames	12,128
7.	South East Thames	10,650
8.	South West Thames	7443
9.	Wessex	6514
10.	Oxford	4306
11.	South Western	7260
12.	West Midlands	12,964
13.	Mersey	8157
14.	North Western	12,882
15.	Scotland	18,119
16.	Wales	8672
17.	Northern Ireland	6470
United Kingdom Total:		160,609

Acute = All Medical and Surgical Specialities and Nuclear Medicine, Pathology and Radiology.

Acute beds reflect the working capacity of the secondary medical and surgical facilities in the NHS, as other services such as operating theatres, central sterile supply departments and X-ray departments are built to accommodate the work flowing through the adjacent wards.

In the case of a nuclear attack, the picture would be entirely different. A completely new clinical situation would arise because of the devastating effects of nuclear explosions both in regard to blast and heat, and also because of the high levels of radiation liberated. These, together with the disruption of communications, rescue and ambulance services, could delay attention to casualties for as long as 10 to 21 days.

During this prolonged period of delay to the commencement of treatment, survivors might die from a wide range of physical, bacteriological, irradiation and psychological causes. Exposure to wet and cold or to heat and fire, would combine with shortages of safe water and food to affect adversely the prospects of survival. Delay in treatment would result in a high incidence of wound infection. Ruptured drainage and sewage systems, together with the presence of decaying corpses and animal carcasses, would increase enormously the hazards of infection. Those already wounded would have the additional problem of radiation sickness from major radioactivity to contend with. The psychological effects of such a disaster can only be conjectured but should not be underestimated.

Major accident schemes existing throughout the country aim at providing high standards of treatment for victims. These schemes are designed to deal with civil disasters in which 25 or more people are injured. This number is insignificant in comparison with the number of casualties resulting even from a solitary 'small' nuclear attack. It is apparent that any schemes in existence would be completely inadequate to deal effectively with such a situation. In a localised attack help from outside the area involved would be restricted by the dangers of moving skilled personnel into an area of irradiation, while evacuation of casualties would produce a similar dilemma. In a major attack medical facilities that survived would be swamped and prove unable to provide acceptable medical care. In these circumstances treatment would consist of only the most simple first-aid measures, with no possibility of complex procedures.

It is unlikely, in the conditions following an attack, that any patient with a third-degree burn involving more than 30 per cent of body surface would survive. Those with more extensive second-degree burns could, however, survive without medical treatment. The plasma and blood requirement for a 50 per cent third degree burn in an adult patient is ten litres in the first 48 hours. It is unlikely that this demand could be met for many, if any, such casualties, even if hospital facilities were available.

Orthopaedic injuries, if severe, would prove fatal and it would be unlikely that the patients themselves would be able to reach medical facilities or receive other than simple first-aid treatment. Spinal injuries would present even greater problems.

Patients with major abdominal and thoracic injuries would be unlikely to survive long enough for effective measures to be taken and survival after this type of injury would be measured in hours.

It appears that the breakdown of specialised medical services would be complete after a major attack and that treatment would be limited to simple first-aid measures and pain relief. The principle of most attention being given to those most likely to survive would replace the former concept that the most seriously ill should receive maximum aid. The Health Service in its present form would disappear after a major nuclear attack on this island.

Medical response to infection in peacetime

Communicable diseases can be counteracted by a variety of medical responses. Mass vaccination programmes can be launched and antibiotics and supportive care are routinely available. After a nuclear attack immunisation programmes would not be feasible. Facilities for diagnosis and treatment of communicable diseases would be largely destroyed. There would not be the resources to deal with more than a fraction of the communicable disease problems which are likely to result. More important than medical treatment for many diseases would be the facilities which sustain modern society, such as food distribution, safe water, shelter, fuel and power supplies. The destruction of these would be particularly conducive to the spread of communicable disease among the population.

Destruction of medical facilities

In Hiroshima 90 per cent of physicians were casualties of the atomic bomb and a similar proportion of nurses were also killed or injured. In the event of another nuclear war it is likely that medical staff and facilities would suffer at least as much if not more than the general population. It has been calculated, for instance, that, in the event of a nuclear attack on London of the same pattern as described in the Home Office's 'Square Leg'[25] exercise in 1980, each surviving doctor would have between 400 and 900 casualties to contend with. If 25 per cent of the population were in the open at the time of the attack each doctor might have to cope with about 175 major burns besides dealing with patients with other injuries. In practice, of course, many casualties would not reach medical help. Most doctors and other health professionals would be unable to render assistance even if they themselves were unharmed because many of the casualties would be in areas of lethal fall-out.

Even a one megaton air-burst bomb over St Paul's Cathedral would result in about 1,600,000 blast injuries (calculated using 1971 census figures for the night-time population). There would probably be about 26,000 major burns if 1 per cent of the population were in the open at the time of the attack and about 650,000 major burns if 25 per cent were out of doors. Casualty figures would be further increased by the many secondary fires which would ensue. It is clear, therefore, that the burden of casualties from just one bomb, dropped on a city, would completely overwhelm the medical facilities of this country. Even in peacetime, Great Britain has only 106 beds specifically for severely burned patients.

Those with major injuries require large quantities of blood as well as monitoring and life support equipment and laboratory facilities. Ideally all major casualties should receive surgical treatment within six hours of injury. Obviously this would be impossible after a nuclear attack. A well-organised surgical team might be able to perform up to seven operations in a 12-hour period under ideal conditions. During a disaster of the magnitude envisaged after a nuclear attack, few surgical teams would be likely to remain intact. Many operating theatres do not carry large reserves of general, abdominal or orthopaedic instruments and delays would occur while instruments were cleaned, packed and autoclaved, even if the necessary public utility services survived.

Many doctors have no recent training in treating patients with trauma and even those who do would probably be reduced to simple procedures such as the reduction of fractures or suturing lacerations, mostly without anaesthesia. Many countries lack recent experience in handling victims of mass disasters. For instance, in the UK between 1951 and 1972 there were only ten disasters involving more than 100 casualties in each.

In order to deal with large numbers of casualties simultaneously the principles of triage were developed. These involve the assessment of each patient by a doctor (or experienced nurse) who assigns them to an appropriate treatment area. In many emergencies even triage would be impossible because of the overwhelming number of casualties resulting from nuclear attack. Hospitals and casualty stations, if not destroyed, are likely to become rallying points for injured survivors and relatives, making organised care even more difficult. In addition, the lack of specific tests for radiation sickness in this situation would further complicate patient assessment.

Four main categories of treatment priorities in military medicine are immediate treatment, delayed treatment, minimal treatment and palliative treatment. The last category comprises those patients who are so severely injured that only complicated or prolonged treatment offers any hope of improving life expectancy. After a nuclear attack, no medical resources could be spent on this group. No drugs which might be of use to survivors would be available for such a purpose. Many people would die without succour.

In peacetime the management of victims of whole-body radiation exposure entails bacteriological monitoring, antibiotics, larninar flow, sterile environment facilities, white cell and platelet transfusion and, in some cases, bone-marrow transplant. These measures would obviously be impossible after a nuclear attack, and there would be essentially no treatment of radiation sickness. Monitoring of the blood-count would not be possible for a meaningful number of patients and therefore medical staff would have no way of determining the extent of radiation exposure until unequivocal clinical evidence of radiation sickness appeared.

Pain relief is likely to be grossly inadequate. Stocks of morphine and other analgesic and anti-emetic drugs would be rapidly exhausted. The quantities of general and local anaesthetics available would likewise be insufficient for the millions of casualties. Many useful drugs would be scattered in neighbourhood pharmacies which would be vulnerable to looting and damage. Hospitals and other medical storage installations would not escape the effects of the attack, and many supplies would be destroyed or inaccessible.

Although it now appears that corpses do not represent the major health threat that was once thought, the presence of large numbers of dead bodies may have severe psychological effects. When United States forces entered Manila[26] in 1944, they faced the problem of burying 39,000 bodies. With few exceptions, troops assigned to this task suffered nausea, vomiting and loss of appetite. Even though local labour was recruited to bury the dead the process still took eight weeks. After a nuclear attack, many bodies would have been vaporised by the thermal effect of the explosions, but vast numbers would still remain to be buried and would be a continual reminder to survivors of the horror that they were experiencing.

Drugs

There would remain the on-going health problems requiring drugs and other long-term care, such as acute illnesses, infections, conditions requiring emergency surgery, malignant disease, chronic conditions (such as diabetes, stroke, chronic bronchitis and arthritis) and conditions which require medical intervention in certain circumstances, such as pregnancy.

Immunisation by vaccines would be particularly difficult. There are very few companies manufacturing vaccines in this country and, if some of these were lost, the lead time for making the product in some other plant might be impossibly long. The manufacture of vaccines within the UK is fairly well centralised in one or two places, but assuming London were a prime target area, a large amount of vaccine would be lost immediately, together with facility to replace it. The Working Party was told that in these circumstances importing would be the answer, given that many drug companies are international and have plant facilities worldwide. However if, as is likely, normal business transactions were to cease, the situation could be hopeless. It was considered that a strategic stockpile was not really a possibility because of cost and the fact that some vaccines deteriorate fairly quickly and would need special storage conditions. Obviously it would be possible to accumulate reserves if the necessary funding were made available.

Given the time scale based on the Home Defence circular, there would be at best a two to three week warning period and then a very short war, during which period drug stocks and drug manufacturing capability would be that of peacetime. It could not be changed during that short warning period. Consequently after a nuclear attack there would remain only whatever was not destroyed of the normal peace requirement. Even in peacetime, however, there is not a particularly large stockpile of drugs. Although it would be possible to encourage stockpiling by buying earlier into the chain, or increasing pharmacy stocks from the requirements of one month to three months, given sufficient notice, it would be expensive. But without such a reserve (and assuming considerable losses during an attack) drug stocks would be low. Very few drugs have a shelf-life of less than 12 months, and some remain viable for three years or more, so there could possibly be a stockpile on a rotating system.

If every hospital increased its supply of drugs by the normal demands of one week, or one month, it would have the advantage that these supplies were dispersed although main hospitals are usually in areas which are vulnerable to attack. Other dispersed storage depots could help solve the problem but would be security risks.

Pain relieving drugs, plasma, blood and intravenous infusions would be in great demand. Many items are made in the hospitals but at least some of these would be destroyed. There are a few manufacturing firms which concentrate on the production of these fluids.

In peacetime stocks of drugs are held by manufacturers and wholesalers. The average manufacturer probably holds something of the order of six weeks' to two months' normal demand in stock, and the wholesaler has perhaps one week's supply. However, some of the more uncommon drug substances might be made by only one manufacturer (who could be the source for the whole world) so it is possible that all of that source could be destroyed. As long as the technology, technical knowledge and equipment were still available, most drugs could be made elsewhere reasonably quickly.

Related to this is the quality of water supplies, which if impaired in volume or purity could lead to problems. Further consideration should be given to the chemicals needed to make contaminated water safe.

Since the Second World War, drug manufacturing has become more centralised and uses much higher technology. The drugs that were available in that war were mainly of vegetable origin—for example quinines, morphines. Ferrotyne, phosphine and sulphonamide were among the few available organic chemicals. Penicillin was not available for clinical use until the Second World War had started. Following the war there was a big expansion of the organic chemical drug substances industry and a movement away from the natural materials.

In general the manufacture of drugs is in two stages. First, there is the manufacture of the drug substance, the active steroid for example. This is done in an organic chemical plant completely different from a pharmaceutical plant (often in a quite different area of technology). By and large, one organic chemical plant is capable of making many substances which could be interchanged. The active drug substance is then compounded into whatever medicament is required, into a tablet or a capsule or into suitable form for injection. This type of work is fairly interchangeable, and again, there should not be great difficulty in switching processes, assuming that staff with the requisite knowledge and the necessary equipment were available. Many international companies hold on file information relating to the manufacture of drugs in a number of countries, so that an attack on one centre would not necessarily result in knowledge of vital processes being lost. Normal secrecy agreements might have to be waived in the event of large-scale disaster.

It is estimated that pharmaceutical companies with their existing facilities could increase their productive capacity by 20 per cent. The bottlenecks would occur in the supply of the ingredients, for example in making synthetic drugs. The precursors of these are often very complex materials in themselves and can originate anywhere in the world. The pharmaceutical industry has not yet been consulted by Government concerning plans to meet the emergency following a nuclear attack.

The only short term way to provide an increased supply of drugs or vaccines is to stockpile at peripheral centres. What happens when this supply is exhausted is an open question. It may be that the main need is water purification. There remains the possibility of a return to herbal remedies which can be obtained from the countryside, as suggested by the East Anglia Regional Health Authority (see Chapter 6). The problem would be to identify and collect the required plants, and to clean them from radioactive fall-out material.

Part B   Calculation of numbers of casualties in a nuclear attack

It is possible to make estimates of the numbers of resulting casualties, given certain assumptions about a set of targets and the weapons used against them, and in the following pages the results of a number of such studies are reported. Those studies submitted to the inquiry concentrate on three of the short-term effects of nuclear explosions: thermal radiation, blast and local fall-out. Since all the weapons would have yields of the order of hundreds of kilotons, or megatons, the effects of initial nuclear radiation are academic, because blast and thermal radiation would be responsible for the immediate deaths and casualties.

In making calculations, the order of effects does not alter the *final* casualty totals. It does, however, have consequences for the intermediate figures calculated for each separate effect, for two reasons. The first is that only 'survivors' of the first effect can be subjected to another effect. The second is that it is probable that victims might be injured in more than one way. Thus of those counted among the burned there will also be some subsequently counted among those receiving mechanical injuries from blast. The same applies for both kinds of injury and serious radiation sickness. In some studies assumptions are made about such combinations of injuries and whether they are likely to result in death. The probability of death from multiple injuries is not simply additive—the injuries are synergistic. Thus, one effect of radiation sickness is to lower the body's resistance to infection; under these conditions, mechanical injuries and burns would be more likely to prove fatal.

It is also possible that individuals might receive the same type of injury from more than one bomb. There is the additional complication that several bombs might fall in the same general area, but at different times. Thus at any given place, the effects might be received repeatedly, and in differing sequences. It is almost impossible to predict what the cumulative consequences for casualties might be. The question of estimating levels of radiation from overlapping fall-out plumes becomes especially complex if the explosions are not more or less simultaneous. Such complications are not usually allowed for, although some of the possible implications are mentioned in the discussion below.

There are several other unpredictable factors involved in such calculations. The results will be affected substantially by the initial assumptions made not only about the targets, but also by the preparedness of the civilian population for attack. Another important variable is the weather, since this can alter the actual effects of weapons; windborne, radioactive debris can travel great distances and can be precipitated with rain as fall-out.

The methods of calculation are approximate. They depend on extrapolations from the effects of the bombs on Hiroshima and Nagasaki, which were very small by today's standards; on the results of various countries' programmes of weapons testing, especially the American above-ground tests of the 1950s and early 1960s; and on theoretical models. In some respects the physical effects of nuclear explosions can be predicted reliably. But since large weapons have never been exploded over cities, or in large numbers simultaneously, and since no nuclear weapons have been used in war since 1945, predictions of the outcome of nuclear explosions in modern conditions must remain highly speculative.

Rotblat (1981)[3] makes some telling points in this connection about the bombs dropped on Hiroshima and Nagasaki. He notes the controversy, discussed in Chapter 1, about the numbers of actual casualties in the two cities. He also draws attention to the fact that the bomb detonated over Nagasaki, although about twice the explosive yield of that on Hiroshima, caused roughly half the number of deaths (see Table 3.2). (Much of the explanation for this lies in the lower population density at Nagasaki.) As Rotblat says:

Thus, even in the only instance in which nuclear weapons were employed against a population, an event which was subsequently investigated very thoroughly, large uncertainties remain about the absolute numbers of casualties; the event also demonstrated that there can be a wide spread in the number of immediate casualties per unit of explosive yield.

Table 3.2. Casualties at Hiroshima and Nagasaki

	Population*	Explosive yield (Mt)	Height of burst (m)	Deaths to end of October 1945
Hiroshima	350,000	0.0125	600	130,000
Nagasaki	270,000	0.022	500	65,000

*At time of explosion, including military and other personnel temporarily present
Source: Hiroshima and Nagasaki (1981)[1] Chapters 2 and 10

Some older American sources give much lower figures, for example:

	Deaths	Injuries
Hiroshima	68,000	76,000
Nagasaki	38,000	21,000

Source: Glasstone and Dolan (eds), *The Effects of Nuclear Weapons* 3rd edn. (1977)[2] p.544 Table 12.09

Calculations of weapons effects and resulting casualties tend to concentrate on those effects which are more easily predicted: blast and, to a lesser extent, short-term fall-out. Those results which are more difficult to estimate, such as fires caused by thermal radiation, or many longer-term consequences of the collapse of the social and technological infrastructure, tend not to be taken into account. As the United States Office of Technology Assessment (1980)[29] remarks in the opening of its study:

The effects of nuclear war that cannot be calculated are at least as important as those for which calculations are attempted. . . . Conservative military planners tend to base their calculations on factors that can be either controlled or predicted, and to make pessimistic assumptions [ie. pessimistic from the attacker's point of view] where control or prediction are impossible. . . . While it is proper for a military plan to provide for the destruction of key targets by the surest means even in unfavourable circumstances, the non-military observer should remember that actual damage is likely to be greater than that reflected in the military calculations. This is particularly true for indirect effects such as deaths resulting from injuries and the unavailability of medical care, or for economic damage resulting from disruption and disorganization rather than from direct destruction.

When numbers of 'survivors' are quoted in quantitative studies, therefore, it should be remembered that these figures represent the short-term survivors of selected effects only. On occasion results are even presented in such a way as to include, without comment, the numbers of 'seriously injured' within the totals of 'survivors'.

The inquiry heard evidence from a number of studies of the effects of hypothetical nuclear attacks on Britain. Most of these are restricted to single cities or limited areas and the computations involved are compiled manually. The inquiry also located some studies of the effects of attack on the country as a whole, for which the calculations were made using computer-based models. In Annex 4 the methods which are generally used for making such estimates are set out in a series of steps.

Casualty estimates for attacks on single cities or limited areas of the UK

The results in terms of casualty estimates of the studies given in evidence to the inquiry are summarised in the following tables (pp.49–51).

Data for Hiroshima and Nagasaki are cited for comparison in Table 3.2.

Table 3.3 summarises studies of attacks on Detroit and Leningrad of varying magnitude, made by the US Office of Technology Assessment (OTA) in *The Effects of Nuclear War* (1980)[29] pp.27–45, again for comparison.

Table 3.4 and 3.5 give the results obtained for scenarios of attack on single cities or limited areas in Britain itself. They comprise:

Table 3.4: an attack on the West Midlands (Birmingham, Wolverhampton and Coventry) with three 1 Mt bombs. (Evidence from A. Qasrawi and others, of the West Midlands branch of Scientists Against Nuclear Arms. This study has been published as *Ground Zero* (1982)[30].)

Table 3.5: an attack on London with 13 Mt. (Evidence from O. Greene, Dr B. Rubin, N. Turok, Dr P. Webber and Dr G. Wilkinson, of the London branch of Scientists Against Nuclear Arms. This study has been published as *London After the Bomb* (1982)[31].)

Casualty estimates for attacks on the UK as a whole

The Working Party received written evidence from the Home Office reporting the predicted effects of different patterns of attack on the country as a whole, in the form of a paper by S. F. J. Butler (then

Table 3.3. US Office of Technology Assessment, *The Effects of Nuclear War* (1980)[29]

Comparative study of nuclear attacks on Detroit and Leningrad (pp.27-45)

	Population	Explosive Yield (Mt)	Height of burst	Blast casualties		Burns casualties	
				Deaths	Injuries	Deaths	Injuries
A Detroit	4,300,000	1	ground	220,000	430,000	1000–190,000	500–75,000
B Detroit	4,300,000	1	air	470,000	630,000		
C Detroit	4,300,000	25	air	1,840,000	1,360,000		
D Leningrad	4,300,000	1	air	890,000	1,260,000		
E Leningrad	4,300,000	9	air	2,460,000	1,100,000		
F Leningrad	4,300,000	$10 \times 0.04 = 0.4$	air	1,020,000	1,000,000		

Assumptions:
No warning, nor sheltering, nor evacuation
Attack at night
Air bursts at a height to maximise 30 psi overpressure contour
Burns casualties (Detroit attack A) range from 3.2 km visibility, 1% of population exposed, to 16 km visibility and 25% exposed.

Table 3.4. Casualties in an attack on the West Midlands

Evidence to BMA Inquiry from A. Qasrawi and West Midlands Branch of Scientists Against Nuclear Arms. Published as *Ground Zero* (1982)[30]

	Population	Explosive Yield (Mt)	Height of burst	Blast casualties		Burns casualties	
				Deaths	Injuries	Deaths	Injuries
Birmingham	1,336,000	1	ground	192,000	422,000	7800–194,000	4800–121,000
Wolverhampton	675,000	1	ground	164,000	210,000	4500–114,000	1000–22,000
Coventry	291,000	1	air	247,000	33,000	500–12,000	0–3000
Totals:	2,302,000	3		603,000	665,000	12,800–320,000	5800–146,000

Assumptions:
Office of Technology Assessment blast casualty criteria
1981 population data estimated by district
Burns casualties assume 19 km visibility, and range from 1% of population exposed to 25% exposed.

Table 3.5. Casualties in an attack on London

Evidence to BMA Inquiry from O. Greene, Dr B. Rubin, N. Turok and Dr P. Webber of Imperial College London, and Dr G. Wilkinson of Reading University, for the London branch of Scientists Against Nuclear Arms. Published as *London After the Bomb* (1982)[31]

Attack pattern:	Explosive yield (Mt)	Height of burst
Heathrow	1	ground
Heathrow	2	air
Croydon	3	ground
Brentford	2	ground
Potters Bar	3	air
Ongar	2	air
	11	

Casualties (out of total population of GLC area of 6,970,000):

Blast casualties		Total fall-out plus blast casualties (after 2 months)		Burns casualties
Deaths	Injuries	Deaths	Injuries	2° and 3° burns
1,135,000	2,481,000	4,503,000–5,351,000	464,000–765,000	50,000+

Assumptions:
OTA blast casualty criteria.
1977 GLC census by boroughs.
No account of overlap of blast areas in counting blast injuries.
Burns casualties assume 1% of population exposed.
Fall-out casualties assume southerly wind 24 km/h; LD 50 for uninjured of 400 rads; LD 50 for injured of 300 rads.
Range of fall-out casualties reflects different assumptions about protective factors of houses in blast damage areas and elsewhere.
Casualties outside GLC area not included.

deputy director of the Home Office Scientific Advisory Branch) entitled 'Scientific Advice in Home Defence'. This paper was delivered at the 1981 meeting of the British Association for the Advancement of Science, and published in C. F. Barnaby and G . P. Thomas (eds), *The Nuclear Arms Race: Control or Catastrophe* (1982)[18]. The Home Office in submitting this paper wished to make clear to the Working Party that it gives 'general background information on scientific support for civil defence, but should not be taken as a definitive source of scientific data nor as an indication of Government policy on protection measures.' It is nevertheless the one publicly available document in which detailed results are presented from the computer model for casualty estimation developed by the Scientific Advisory Branch (now the Research and Development Branch).

The attack scenarios adopted by Butler, and the corresponding casualty estimates, are set out in Table 3.6. Butler illustrates the example of an attack with 179 weapons totalling 193 megaton (Mt) on a mixture of military targets and cities (not individually specified). This is shown as attack A in the Table. He also shows the predicted effects of an alternative series of patterns of attack (B, C and D in the Table), which are taken to be directed respectively against 'primarily military targets', 'military targets plus population centres' and 'primarily civilian targets'. In each case the results are shown for an attack with 84 weapons totalling 181 Mt, in which the population is either assumed to be at home (corresponding to the official 'stay-put' policy as promulgated through the *Protect and Survive* leaflet)[32], or else is 'dispersed' according to some policy of evacuation.

Casualty totals are also shown for cases B, C and D (and with a 'stay-put' population) for much greater total weights of attack: 500 Mt and 3000 Mt.

In addition there are some indications given of the consequences for the results of attack A of altering various assumptions relating to blast and fall-out casualty rates, which will be discussed further below.

It is interesting to note the *average* yield of weapon envisaged by the Home Office in the 193 Mt and 181 Mt patterns of attack. These are 1.08 and 2.15 Mt respectively.

Other studies of the effects of attack at a national scale have also been made by S. Openshaw of Newcastle University and P. Steadman of the Open University, using their own computer model. These have been reported in a series of papers: 'On the geography of a worst case nuclear attack on the population of Britain', *Political Geography Quarterly* July 1982[15], 263–278; 'Predicting the consequences of a nuclear attack on Britain: models, results and public policy implications', *Environment and Planning C*[33], in press; 'On the geography of the bomb', paper delivered to the 1983 conference of the Institute of British Geographers[20].

The results are illustrated in Table 3.7. The first of these studies[15] is a 'worst case' attack scenario on cities, shown as attack A in the Table. This is a somewhat artificial calculation relating to the blast effects only of 1 Mt air-burst bombs on cities. It is made as follows: the computer

Table 3.6. Casualties in various attacks on the United Kingdom

Estimates by the Home Office Scientific Advisory Branch, reported in S. F. J. Butler, 'Scientific Advice in Home Defence' in C. F. Barnaby and G. P. Thomas (eds) (1982) *The Nuclear Arms Race: Control or Catastrophe*[18] pp.135-163

Total population of UK (1971) census: 56 million

			Casualties (millions)			
Attack pattern	No. of weapons	Explosive yield (Mt)	Killed or trapped*	Fall-out deaths	All deaths	Seriously injured
A. Military targets and cities	129 air-burst 50 ground-burst ——— 179	84 109 ——— 193	} 16	'under 1'	17	3.5
			Total deaths (blast plus fall-out) rise to 26.9 million with 'more severe blast criterion'			

			Total *deaths* (blast plus fall-out, millions)	
	No. of weapons	Explosive yield (Mt)	'Stay-put'† population	'Dispersed' population
B. Primarily military targets	84 NA NA	181 500 3000	5.6 13.4 43.1	4.5
C. Military targets and population centres	84 NA NA	181 500 3000	15.7 23.5 47.6	6.7
D. Primarily civilian targets	84 NA NA	181 500 3000	19 39.2 50.4	7.3

Assumptions:

*Those 'trapped' are assumed to die

†The population is assumed in general to be at home, following the official 'stay-put' policy. However, the results are shown for cases B, C and D above, with the 181 Mt attack, of a 'dispersed' pattern of population distribution, resulting from a programme of evacuation.

Casualty estimates, especially fall-out casualties, assume 'general adherence to *Protect and Survive*[32] advice'.

There is no specific blast shelter provision.

Table 3.7. Casualties in various attacks on the United Kingdom

Estimates by Dr S. Openshaw of Newcastle University and P. Steadman of the Open University, reported in 'On the geography of a worst case nuclear attack on the population of Britain', *Political Geography Quarterly*, July 1982, 263–278; 'Predicting the consequences of a nuclear attack on Britain: models, results and public policy implications', *Environment and Planning C*, in press; 'On the geography of the bomb', paper delivered to 1983 conference of Institute of British Geographers.

Total population of UK excluding N. Ireland (1971 census): 54 million.

Attack pattern	No. of weapons	Explosive yield (Mt)	*Deaths* from blast effects only (millions)*
A. 'Worst case' attacks on population			
10 cities	10 air burst	10	6.2-12
50 cities	50 air burst	50	17 -26.7
100 towns and cities	100 air burst	100	24.6-35.1
200 towns and cities	200 air burst	200	33.1-43.3

B. 1980 'Square Leg' exercise (military targets and cities)

No. of weapons	Explosive yield (Mt)	Casualties (millions)				
		Burns deaths	Blast deaths	Fall-out deaths	All deaths	Seriously injured
58 air-burst	88.5 ⎫					
67 ground-burst	108 ⎬	2.5	13	11.2	26.7	6.8
125	196.5 ⎭					

C. 'Counterforce' attack primarily on military, with some industrial targets

119 air-burst	82 ⎫					
221 ground-burst	140 ⎬	3.1	20.2	15.3	38.6	4.3
340	222 ⎭					

Assumptions:

OTA blast casualty criteria throughout.

*Ranges of blast deaths in attack A correspond to the two assumptions, either that all seriously injured survive (even if injured by blast more than once), or that all seriously injured die.

Burns casualties assume 5% of population exposed. Fall-out casualties assume wind speed 24 km/h, southerly in attack B, south-south-westerly in attack C; LD 50 of 450 rads. National average protective factor of houses is 8 for areas without blast damage, and reduced in blast-affected areas depending on peak overpressures. Those 'seriously injured' from two or more causes are assumed to die. Use of census data implies a night-time 'at home' distribution of population.

searches the entire country for that target where the total number of killed and injured by blast is the greatest. This, as one would expect, is in central London. Those calculated as dead are removed from the population data base, and the same process is repeated to find the second worst target, and so on, up to 200 bombs. The targets so selected follow in their distribution, naturally enough, a population density map of the country. Cumulative casualties are given in the Table for 10, 50, 100 and 200 Mt.

It is obvious that this is not a militarily plausible pattern of attack as such. The exercise does, however, serve to do two things: to show the very worst possible consequences with respect to blast casualties (for this size of bomb) at a national level, as a benchmark against which more realistic scenarios can be measured; and to identify in order of seriousness those individual targets, over the whole country, where blast casualties would be most numerous. The ranges of figures for blast deaths given in Table 3.7 relate to two different assumptions: at the most pessimistic that all those counted as injured would subsequently die, and, at the most optimistic, that all those counted as injured would survive (even though many would be injured by blast from more than one bomb). A reasonable figure would therefore lie somewhere between these extremes.

Openshaw and Steadman have further used their model to investigate two scenarios of attack (reported in the *Environment and Planning*[33] and Institute of British Geographers papers[20]) which are strategically more plausible. The first (Attack B in the Table) is the 1980 'Square Leg' exercise which combines military targets and cities. In this 125 weapons are used with a total yield of 196.5 Mt, giving an average yield per bomb of 1.57 Mt.

A second scenario (C in the Table) is a 'counterforce' attack pattern which is directed principally at targets of military significance with some industrial targets also included. It is the scenario described previously in Chapter 2, and differs from the Home Office studies and 'Square Leg' by taking warheads with explosive yields corresponding to those of actual Soviet weapons. This accounts for the total megatonnage (222 Mt) being made up from a large number (340) of relatively low-yield warheads (average 0.65 Mt).

Totals are shown for predicted burns, blast and fall-out deaths, and for numbers seriously injured from all causes. It should be appreciated that these three effects are considered by the computer model in this same sequence, and that those counted as seriously injured from burns may subsequently be killed by blast effects and so on. The final total for casualties thus represents only those who survive injuries from any one of the three causes. (If they are counted as seriously injured from two or more causes, they are assumed to die.)

All these results can be used to illustrate the uncertainties of calculation already referred to, as well as to show some of the consequences of varying the initial conditions assumed in an attack scenario. It will be immediately evident from Tables 3.6 and 3.7, for example, that big differences can occur in the total casualties predicted for a similar weight and pattern of attack. Compare attack A in Table 3.6 with attack B in Table 3.7; both are on mixed military and city targets, with around 195 Mt. However, predicted total casualties are 20.5 million in the former and 33.5 million in the latter. Some explanations for such enormous differences will be discussed below.

Discussion of uncertainties and variable factors in casualty estimates

Population distribution

If warning were given of an attack, and if sufficient time were available, it might be possible to evacuate people from places thought to be at risk. In the absence of an official evacuation policy, people might try to move to what they perceived to be safer areas on their own initiative. The use of census data in the calculations assumes people to stay at home. The Home Office relates the use of census data in its computer model to the current British 'stay-put' policy, by which householders are encouraged to stay in their own areas, and no official plans exist for evacuation (although this policy is presently under review). Butler[18] nevertheless shows results, as mentioned, for a modified distribution of the population, dispersed more uniformly across the country. The result, for a combined attack on military targets and population centres with 181 Mt (Attack C in Table 3.6), is for the estimated total number of deaths (from blast effects and fall-out) to drop by some 9 million. The effect is even more marked than this where primarily 'civilian targets' are attacked, less so when mostly military targets are chosen.

The census furthermore records the distribution of the population at *night-time*. If city centres were to be attacked without warning during working hours then it is likely that many more casualties would result than would be predicted using census figures.

For Britain the 1971 census is available by one-kilometre grid squares throughout the country. Both the Home Office and Openshaw/Steadman models use this data. The 1981 figures are not yet fully released. Some non-computer studies introduce approximations by using figures for population density averaged over larger area units.

The higher the density of population, the greater the number of casualties caused by a given size of bomb. This is illustrated by the OTA's calculation (Table 3.3) for 1 Mt air-burst weapons on Detroit and Leningrad. The blast casualties for Leningrad are almost twice those for Detroit as a direct consequence of higher housing densities in Leningrad. A great part of the difference between the Hiroshima and Nagasaki casualties can be attributed to this same cause. Glasstone and Dolan (1977)[2] quote average densities of 8500 and 5800 persons per square mile for Hiroshima and Nagasaki respectively (p.544). (These absolute figures may be open to question in the light of more recent analysis; nonetheless, for the point at issue it is the comparative densities which are important.) The difference in density was particularly marked in the zones between 0.6 and 1.6 miles from ground zero in the two cities.

Explosive yields and heights of burst of weapon

As discussed in Chapter 1, the range of blast effects of a nuclear explosion is not directly proportional to yield, but only to the cube root of the yield. Thus for an 8 Mt ground-burst bomb, the radius for a given peak overpressure contour would be only twice that for a 1 Mt ground-burst. The area affected would thus be four times greater. The consequences for casualties are indicated in the OTA studies[29]. Increasing the yield of bombs on Detroit from 1 Mt to 25 Mt (both air-burst) results in only a threefold increase in total blast casualties. There is the further consideration that the size of any city is finite and the number of casualties obviously cannot exceed the total population. Such a 'law of diminishing returns' is beginning to operate in the case of Detroit. Similar effects are illustrated by the comparison of 1 Mt and 9 Mt air-bursts on Leningrad. Even in terms of the logic (if there is any) of nuclear war, weapons of the order of size of 10 or 20 Mt seem to make little military sense.

An important corollary is that blast casualties caused by a single bomb may be fewer than the total for a number of weapons whose combined yield is not so great as the one bomb. This is shown by the OTA examples for Leningrad of a 1 Mt air-burst, as against ten 40-kiloton air-bursts. The number of blast casualties is roughly the same in both cases, although the total yield of the ten weapons is only 0.4 Mt. There is no comfort to be taken therefore from any possible trend towards lower-yield weapons in the world's strategic arsenals, so long as the total yield used in an attack is not correspondingly reduced.

This is a point which we will take up again in discussing the effects of attack on the country as a whole.

The number of blast casualties for a ground-burst bomb is much smaller than for an air-burst bomb (exploded at 'optimum height') of equal yield. This follows directly from the reduced range of blast effects for ground-bursts as discussed in Chapter 1. The OTA's 1 Mt ground-burst on Detroit causes roughly half the number of blast casualties of the 1 Mt air-burst. It is ground-bursts on the other hand which are principally responsible for radioactive fall-out and for delayed casualties due to ionising radiation.

It is clear that bombs even of high yield dropped on military targets will not cause enormous numbers of blast or burns casualties if the immediately surrounding areas are lightly populated. By contrast, at the opposite end of the scale, it is possible for a single 1 Mt air-burst bomb dropped on a city centre to cause more than a million casualties from blast alone. This is illustrated in the OTA case study of Detroit. The evidence for Birmingham (Table 3.4) gives blast casualties of 600,000 for a bomb targeted on the M6/A38(M) interchange ('Spaghetti Junction'). Openshaw and Steadman's 'worse case' analysis indicates that for a slightly different ground zero in Birmingham this number could rise to over a million, and that five such other targets exist in Britain (in Manchester, Glasgow, Liverpool and in east and west London).

The blast casualties quoted for Leningrad by the OTA for a 1 Mt air-burst exceed two million. Openshaw and Steadman's single worst bomb, on central London, causes more than three million blast casualties. In this context it is important to notice that the study for London summarised in Table 3.5 takes the targets selected for the 'Square Leg' exercise — and that all of these are in the outer suburbs, none in the centre of the city.

Ranges of blast overpressure

The convention of representing the zones affected by blast around a nuclear explosion as perfectly circular assumes absolutely flat ground. The same applies to the areas exposed to given levels of thermal radiation. In practice the shapes of hills and valleys would create shadows, modifying the ranges of damage — though in ways which would be hard to predict in detail. (The fact that Nagasaki is sited in a valley had a substantial effect in elongating the damage areas, by comparison with the roughly circular zone devastated at Hiroshima.) Otherwise, the ranges of blast overpressure for a specified height and yield of burst are thought to be reliably predictable.

There are nevertheless some substantial discrepancies between figures from American sources, and those quoted in certain Home Office documents. The Working Party received evidence on this point from P. Steadman of the Open University. The issue is also discussed in *London After the Bomb*[31] (p.14 and Table 2).

The standard authority on blast and indeed most other effects of nuclear weapons is Glasstone and Dolan (eds) (1977)[2], which was prepared for the US Departments of Defence and Energy. Most work on the estimation of casualties in hypothetical patterns of attack relies on this source for basic weapons effects data. This is true of all the studies reported here, including those by the Home Office. The book is issued by the Home Office to its regional scientific advisers, and is used as the basis for calculating the physical effects of blast in the Home Office computer model, as described by Bentley (1981)[34]. It is important to emphasise right at the outset that the Home Office casualty figures from Butler (1982)[18], reproduced here in Table 3.6, are *not* it seems affected by these discrepancies, despite the fact that Butler actually illustrates in his paper (Fig. 4) blast effects data which differ substantially from Glasstone and Dolan.

Home Office practice is to define four concentric damage rings, labelled, A, B, C and D from ground zero outwards. The outer edges of these rings correspond to peak overpressure values of 11, 6, 1.5 and 0.75 psi respectively. Taking the example of a 1 Mt ground burst, Table 3.8 compares radii for these rings according to Glasstone and Dolan on the one hand, and Home Office sources, specifically *Nuclear Weapons* (1974)[35] p.33 Table 9, and *Domestic Nuclear Shelters: Technical Guidance* (1981)[17] p.9, Fig. 6, on the other hand. Distances are converted to kilometres throughout.

The radii of the A and B rings, where damage is heaviest and casualties most numerous, are somewhat greater according to Glasstone and Dolan. Since these are the radii of circular damage areas, the

Table 3.8. 1 Mt ground-burst

| Ring | Peak over-pressure (psi) | Radius (km) | |
		Home Office	Glasstone
A	11	2.5	3
B	6	3.5	4
C	1.5	9	9
D	0.75	14	14

discrepancy is quite significant. It increases the area of the A ring from
20 km^2 (Home Office) to 28 km^2 (Glasstone); and the area of A and B
rings together from 38 km^2 (Home Office) to 50 km^2 (Glasstone).
Comparable discrepancies are found for weapons of other explosive
yields. The Home Office agreed in evidence to the Working Party that
these differences occur, but said that: 'It is not possible to discuss in
every case which is "correct", as the range for a given overpressure may
be influenced by a number of factors.'

For *air-bursts*, the discrepancies are much greater. The Home Office's
Nuclear Weapons (1974)[35] states (p.35): 'For practical purposes it can be
assumed that the ranges of various categories of damage for ground-
burst bombs . . . would be increased by 30 per cent if the same sized
weapon were air-burst near the optimum height.' This relationship, of
an increase of 30 per cent in range for air-bursts, is reiterated in
Domestic Nuclear Shelters: Technical Guidance (1981)[17] p.9 Fig. 6. The
resulting radii for a 1 Mt bomb are given in Table 3.9. They correspond
very closely to those cited by Butler (1982)[18] p.144 Fig. 4, in his
account of the method used for casualty estimation on the Home Office
computer model. They may be compared again with equivalent figures
calculated from data in Glasstone and Dolan (1977)[2]

Table 3.9. 1 Mt air-burst

Ring	Peak over-pressure (psi)	Radius (km)	
		Home Office	Glasstone
A	11	3.25	4.25
B	6	4.55	6
C	1.5	11.7	14.5
D	0.75	18.2	24 approx.

Instead of an increase in radius of 30 per cent over ground-bursts,
these figures from Glasstone and Dolan amount to an increase of more
like 50 or 60 per cent. In this example, the American data are for a burst
whose height is such as to maximise the area affected at the 10 psi (or
greater) overpressure level, which would be a usual order of figure to
take. The height of burst for these published Home Office figures is not
specified. For bombs detonated at heights to maximise different damage
levels the radii as given by Glasstone and Dolan would alter
appreciably, although large overall discrepancies would still remain.
The discrepancies apply equally to radii scaled for explosive yields
other than one megaton.

Clearly, the addition of 30 per cent to the ranges for an equivalent yield ground-burst weapon is intended by the Home Office as an approximation. Nevertheless it results in very substantial differences in the areas of all four damage rings, as Table 3.10 indicates:

Table 3.10. Blast damage areas for 1 Mt air burst

Damage rings	Area (km²)	
	Home Office	Glasstone
A	33	57
A + B	65	113
A + B + C	430	660
A + B + C + D	1040	1800 approx.

For the zones subjected to the heaviest damage (the A and B rings, where the Home Office expects the majority of casualties to occur) the areas according to the American figures are nearly double those given by the Home Office.

Questioned by the Working Party on this point, the Home Office representative said that the rule of adding 30 per cent to the range for a ground burst '. . . is too great a simplification for many practical applications (as well as 1.3 being a rather atypical factor) and it may have originated in the early days when detailed information on weapon effects was inhibited by security restrictions . . . It is unfortunate that the old 30 per cent rule has been re-quoted (even though it is only intended to serve as a general indication and is not actually applied in any calculation) in *Domestic Nuclear Shelters: Technical Guidance*[17] and in S. F. J. Butler's paper[18].' The Home Office re-emphasised that Glasstone and Dolan (1977)[2] is currently used in all casualty estimation work and in the computer model.

Blast casualty rates

In order to relate the physical characteristics of the blast wave from a nuclear explosion to estimates of resulting casualties, it is necessary to derive some set of relationships between different ranges of peak overpressure value, and the percentages of the population killed or injured in the corresponding zones. The relationships are not simple, since blast casualties can be caused in a variety of ways—by the collapse of buildings, by people being propelled at speed into obstacles, or being hit by flying projectiles as described earlier. It seems that the blast casualty models which have been proposed by different authors rely in part on such statistics as exist for the Japanese victims, in part on evidence from experiments with animal cadavers, and in part on the results of the American programme of weapons tests (in which, for example, test buildings were constructed at varying distances from ground zero with monitoring of the damage caused).

The Office of Technology Assessment (OTA) uses in its study[29] the relationships shown in Table 3.11. It describes these assumptions as 'relatively conservative'. They relate to the entire population present in the respective zones, regardless of whether people are in or out of doors. (They do, however, refer to houses and other buildings above ground. If some fraction of the population had access to special-purpose blast-proof shelters, these figures would not apply.) According to the OTA, a typical house would be collapsed by an overpressure of about 5 psi. 'The calculations used here assume a mean lethal overpressure of 5 to 6 psi for people in residences, meaning that more than half of those whose houses are blown down on top of them will nevertheless survive.'

Table 3.11. 'Vulnerability of population in various overpressure zones' US Office of Technology Assessment, *The Effects of Nuclear War* Fig. 1 p.19

Overpressure range (psi)	% Dead	% Injured
Greater than 12	98	2
5–12	50	40
2–5	5	45
1–2	0	25

The Working Party was informed that these blast casualty rates were obtained in turn from the US Department of Defense (who have a series of standard factors) since the OTA thought it important for the credibility of their results to use assumptions about weapons effects similar to those of the Defense Department. (Glasstone and Dolan do not give precise figures for blast casualty rates.) The principle source for the OTA rates, it seems, is analysis of the American weapons tests conducted prior to the 1963 nuclear test-ban treaty.

Other American studies use a simpler method of calculation. They assume that the number of people killed by blast outside the 5 psi contour is equal to the number of survivors inside, and thus that the number of deaths will equal the number of people inside the 5 psi range. For a uniform population density this gives slightly more fatalities than the OTA model.

All the studies summarised in Tables 3.4–3.7 use these OTA blast casualty rates, with the sole exception of that by the Home Office. Here again there are large discrepancies between the Home Office assumptions and those of the Americans. The Working Party received evidence on this subject again from P. Steadman, from the *London After the Bomb*[31] group, and from J. Marrow, Consultant in Accident and Emergency Care at Birkenhead General Hospital.

The assumptions about blast casualty rates made by the Home Office are indicated only in rather general terms in Butler's paper (Fig. 4, p.144):

A ring: 'Fatality level could exceed 85 per cent without blast shelter protection'

B ring: 'Fatality level could exceed 40 per cent without blast shelter protection'

C ring: 'Blast could cause lethal flying missiles'

In *Domestic Nuclear Shelters: Technical Guidance*[17] (Fig. 6, p.9), probable levels of blast casualties are again given broadly as:

A ring: 'High probability of death or serious injury'

B ring: 'About 10 per cent killed; 35 per cent trapped; others injured'

C ring: 'About 25 per cent trapped or seriously injured at inner edge of ring'

D ring: 'No deaths; few injuries expected'

However, the Home Office representative confirmed in evidence to the Working Party that both these sets of statements refer to a more precise set of casualty assumptions in current use, which are built into the 'Weapons Effects Computers' (circular slide-rules) issued to Home Office scientific advisers. These figures go back in turn to casualty rates published under the title 'Exercise ARC', reproduced here as Figure 3.1. 'Exercise ARC' gives three continuous curves for '% killed', '% trapped' and '% untrapped—seriously injured'. These are related in effect to peak overpressure values (shown in the figure as ranges for ground-burst bombs of different yields). The Home Office in calculating total casualties in an attack assumes that those counted as 'trapped' will subsequently die.

Figure 3.2 shows for comparison the blast casualty rates adopted variously by the Home Office (above) and the Office of Technology Assessment (below) for a 1 Mt air-burst bomb. In both cases the overpressure ranges are taken from Glasstone and Dolan (1977)[2]. The difference is clearly very marked indeed. If a uniform density of

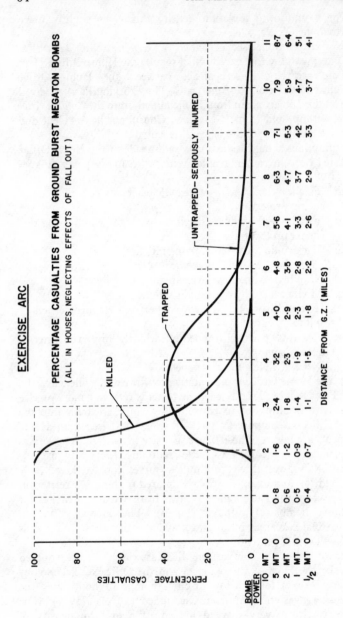

Figure 3.1. Home Office blast casualty rates. Those 'trapped' are generally assumed to die
Source: Home Office (1959) p.10

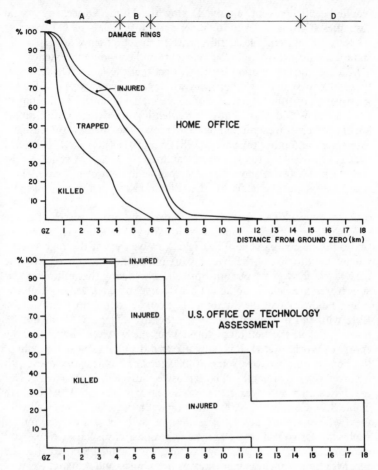

Figure 3.2. Blast casualties for a 1 Mt air-burst detonated at 2200 metres, according to the Home Office (above) and the US Office of Technology Assessment (below)

population is assumed, then the total killed according to the OTA model is roughly twice the figure given by the Home Office (assuming all those 'trapped' are to die).

For the numbers injured there is evidently a huge discrepancy. For the greater part of the C damage ring, total casualties according to the Home Office are below 5 per cent, whereas according to the OTA they would be 50 per cent. In the D ring the Home Office expects no casualties at all, whereas in the inner part of this zone the OTA expect 25 per cent injured. These differences in the outer rings are especially significant since they apply to circular areas of considerable extent.

Much of the explanation lies in the fact that the Home Office derive these blast casualty rates not from studies of nuclear weapons for the most part, but from experience of conventional chemical explosions in the Second World War. Thus P. R. Bentley in a Home Office report 'Blast overpressure and fall-out radiation dose models for casualty assessment and other purposes' (1981)[34] remarks (p.4) that: 'In World War II fatalities due to blast started at an overpressure of about 3.5 psi and reached 100% at about 40 psi for people in their own homes.' This relationship approximately fits the killed plus trapped curve in Figure 3.2.

Glasstone and Dolan, however, remark in several places that the effects of conventional chemical explosions and nuclear explosions are by no means comparable. They say: '. . . because of the high energy yields, the duration of the overpressure (and winds) associated with the blast wave, for a given peak overpressure, is so long that injuries occur at overpressures which would not be effective in a chemical explosion.'

Some indication of the difference is given by comparing deaths in the Blitz with deaths caused by the two bombs in Japan. About 60,000 people died in the bombings throughout the whole of Britain in the course of World War II. It is estimated that the total explosive weight of the bombs dropped was some 70,000 tons. Thus roughly one death occurred per ton of bombs. The explosive equivalent in tons of TNT of the Hiroshima and Nagasaki bombs together was 35,000 (compare Table 3.2). Certainly 100,000 and perhaps more than 200,000 died in the two cities; this gives between three and six deaths per ton of explosive. Of course, there are many reasons why such a simple and crude calculation is misleading (although it should be noted that the Japanese figures include many deaths from burns and radiation, as well as from blast effects). But it serves to give some notion of the much greater potential for damage and injury of nuclear weapons, aside from their vastly magnified power in simple explosive equivalent.

Questioned on these discrepancies by the Working Party, the Home Office representative said:

The original blast damage/injury rules used by the Home Office were derived from the results of a study by members of the British Mission to Japan[36] of blast damage to buildings at Hiroshima and Nagasaki, combined with an analysis of casualty rates in the then typical UK houses with various degrees of high explosive (HE) bomb damage. These rules represented the only information of its kind that was available for official use for some years. It has often been suggested that they might underestimate casualties from megaton range weapons on account of the possibly severer effects of the longer duration blast wave. Over recent years, note has been taken of the changes occurring in UK house construction, and of recent research carried out in the USA. Currently this Branch [Scientific Advisory Branch] is as a priority item in its Civil Defence Research programme reviewing the blast damage/injury rules with the aim of producing a revised set of rules that are more soundly based and applicable to the current UK situation. The Branch has good liaison with the USA experts in this field, and a considerable amount of research information has already been secured, and more is promised. However, the subject is a complex one, and results for the UK are not expected quickly.

In the context of the reference here to the British Mission to Japan, it is interesting to compare the data for death rates in the two cities by distance from ground zero, as given in the Mission's report, *The Effects of the Atomic Bombs at Hiroshima and Nagasaki* (1946)[36] p.21, with what the current Home Office casualty rates would predict for Hiroshima. The respective curves are illustrated in Figure 3.3. In the latter case the overpressure ranges are calculated using Glasstone and Dolan, assuming a 12.5 Mt yield at 600 metres altitude. The British Mission's death rates are comparable with those given by more recent studies, both American and Japanese.

As for the OTA blast casualty assumptions, these scale quite well to the Japanese data, although there are a number of problems involved besides the uncertainties over the actual casualty figures. There is the fact that the OTA rates refer only to blast deaths and injuries, while casualties are not distinguished by cause in the Japanese figures — although as many as 70 per cent of casualties who survived suffered blast injuries, and this proportion was probably higher among those who died. There is also the problem that the OTA casualty rates are presumably intended to apply to weapons in the megaton range and to modern American house construction.

On this latter point, the Home Office representative told the Working Party that

. . . the casualty rules adopted in the OTA report 'Effects of Nuclear War' should not as they stand be taken as directly applicable to the UK. Not only are they too broad to be of use for many analyses, but they are based on data relating to USA house construction (it would appear wood frame) and incorporate arbitrary assumptions for the distribution of persons around houses, and their posture. Thus the OTA rules are likely to be unduly severe for assessments of attacks on the UK.

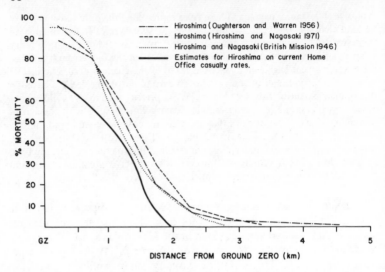

Figure 3.3. Death rates (all causes) at Hiroshima and Nagasaki by distance from ground zero

The dotted line shows figures combined for both cities, according to the British Mission to Japan (1946) p.21. The broken lines show figures for Hiroshima given by Oughterson and Warren (1956) p.30, and in *Hiroshima and Nagasaki* (1971) p.113.

The solid line shows what current Home Office casualty rates would predict for Hiroshima. (Those 'trapped' are counted as dead. Blast overpressure ranges are calculated from Glasstone and Dolan (1977) assuming a 12.5 kt burst at 600 metres.)

The point about differing house construction between the UK and the USA seems open to question, however, since as mentioned the OTA calculations are based on the assumption that a typical house will be collapsed by an overpressure of 5 psi. Glasstone and Dolan (pp.178–184) report weapons tests with actual buildings at the Nevada test site in the 1950s, which showed that standard American wood-frame houses were demolished by about 4 psi, and that houses with brick and cinder block walls, similar to much recent British house construction, were destroyed by 5 psi. On trends in British house design since the 1940s, it would seem that these have been if anything towards lighter and less blast-resistant construction. Certainly multi-storey buildings, prefabricated structures and buildings incorporating large areas of glazing would seem to be particularly vulnerable.

In Butler's[18] illustrations of Home Office casualty estimates for attacks on the United Kingdom, the consequences are shown of applying a 'more severe blast criterion' (see Table 3.6). For Attack A with 179 weapons totalling 193 Mt, the effect is to raise total blast deaths to some 27 million, from a figure of 16 million for the 'standard current casualty model'. The Home Office representative told the Working Party that this 'more severe blast criterion' was not directly related to, but was in fact not far different from, the OTA assumptions.

Burns caused by direct thermal radiation

All of the studies summarised in Tables 3.4, 3.5 and 3.7 (Attacks B and C) make estimates of numbers who would suffer burns by direct exposure to thermal radiation from the nuclear explosion. Each of them follow broadly the methods of calculation set out by the OTA in *The Effects of Nuclear War*[29] (pp.31-32). The OTA assumes that: '. . . exposure to more than 6.7 cal/cm^2 produces eventual death, and exposure to more than 3.4 cal/cm^2 produces a significant injury, requiring specialized medical treatment.' This implies that for a one megaton explosion, third- and second-degree burns would be fatal, while first-degree burns would be serious enough to require medical attention.

Glasstone and Dolan[2] make slightly less pessimistic assumptions. They indicate that, under the conditions of nuclear war, people suffering third degree burns would certainly die, and that people with second-degree burns would need medical treatment to survive, especially if they were suffering radiation sickness at the same time.

J. Marrow in evidence to the Working Party questioned the OTA figures:

. . . the amount of heat energy required to cause burning is not altogether clear. *The Effects of Nuclear War* makes the assumption that at least 3.4 cal/cm^2 of heat energy falling on skin would be sufficient to produce significant burning. Experimental work as far back as 1956 (Butterfield et al., 'Flash burns from atomic weapons' *Surgery, Gynaecology and Obstetrics* (1956)[37] 103, 6, 655-665) suggested that 2.0 cal/cm^2 would be sufficient to burn 50% of those exposed to it. If smaller amounts of heat are needed to inflict burning, then burns would occur at a considerably greater range, from any given weapon.

Assuming some relation can be established between thermal radiation exposure and seriousness of resulting burns, there are two further factors which can have very large effects on estimated numbers of burns casualties. The first is atmospheric visibility, which determines the ranges at which varying levels of exposure to radiation are experienced. In an example given by the OTA: 'When visibility is 10 miles (16 km), a 1-Mt [ground-burst] explosion produces second-degree burns at a distance of 6 miles (10 km), while under circumstances when visibility is 2 miles (3 km), the range of second-degree burns is only 2.7 miles (4.3 km).'

On the other hand, the ranges would be *increased* somewhat if there were cloud cover above most of the fireball, or snow cover on the ground, both of which would reflect the heat flash.

The second factor is the percentage of the population exposed (i.e. in direct line of sight to the fireball). This fraction could vary greatly with time of day, with the weather and time of year, and in particular with the fact of warning of an attack, since with thermal radiation, unlike blast effects, it is possible to take precautions by sheltering inside buildings. For illustration the OTA takes extreme values for visibility of two miles (3.2 km) and ten miles (16 km), and for percentage of population exposed, one per cent and 25 per cent. The resulting casualties for the case of a 1 Mt ground-burst on Detroit (Table 3.3) range from 1000 killed and 500 injured in the most favourable circumstances to 190,000 killed and 75,000 injured in the worst case.

The hypothetical attack on the West Midlands analysed by Qasrawi *et al.*[30] (Table 3.4) follows the OTA in taking between one per cent and 25 per cent exposed, and assumes a clear atmosphere and 19 km visibility. The numbers calculated as killed by direct burns vary between 12,800 and 320,000, and the numbers seriously injured between 5,800 and 146,000. Of this figure of 146,000, some 18 per cent are calculated as suffering combined injuries from burns and blast effects.

In the national studies by Openshaw and Steadman (Table 3.7) the figures quoted for burns deaths assume five per cent exposed, and again clear visibility with a range of 19 km. In Attack B ('Square Leg') burns deaths total 2.5 million and burns injuries 0.9 million; in Attack C, burns deaths total 3.1 million and burns injuries 1.2 million. With 25 per cent of the population exposed, the casualties in Attack B would rise by more than another two million. Openshaw and Steadman have also experimented with Glasstone and Dolan's as well as the OTA burns casualty assumptions. The difference for five per cent exposed in the 'Square Leg' attack is about a quarter of a million more burns deaths and injuries for the OTA criteria than those assumed by Glasstone and Dolan.

The Home Office casualty model by contrast omits any consideration of burns, caused either directly by exposure to the fireball, or indirectly by fires. This accounts for the absence of burns casualties in Butler's illustrations of Home Office estimates in Table 3.6. In evidence to the

Working Party the Home Office explained these omissions on the grounds that:

. . . we assume (a) that the population is warned in accordance with arrangements for warning the population of nuclear attack and that they have heeded advice to get under cover, and (b) that there would be no casualties attributable *directly* to fire unless there were a conflagration or a firestorm. The occurrence of either is a possibility, but the probability of occurrence in the UK situation is thought to be small and no reliable data are available to us which justify their inclusion. However, the question is not closed, and a need for studies may arise in which assumptions relating to exposure to thermal flash, and to the effects of fires would have to be made. There is also a possibility that at some future date results of new research may allow the inclusion of fire casualties in routine assessments.

The Home Office's current assumptions in relation to direct burns thus imply not only that warning of an attack is available and that this warning reaches the whole population, but also that people taking cover indoors remain sheltered. This would not apply in circumstances where blast damage was caused by one weapon, and people then emerged— perhaps to help in rescue work or to prepare fall-out shelters—only to be exposed to a second weapon.

All the studies cited, British and American, take no account of any additional burns cases caused indirectly by fires. However, attempts to calculate fire damage to property and possible resulting casualties are generally excluded not because these would not occur, but because of the problems of estimation. As the OTA says: 'the extent of fire damage depends on factors such as weather and details of building construction that make it much more difficult to predict than blast damage.'

Another doubtful question is to what extent survivors, especially the injured, would be able either to escape or to control fires. It is perhaps improbable that much effective fire-fighting effort could be organised, given the likelihood of water mains being broken, appliances destroyed, and roads blocked. On the other hand the Home Office view, according to Butler, is that: 'the possibility of widespread fires could be greatly reduced by suitable precautions and by the control of incipient fires by survivors of the attack.'

Radiation levels from local fall-out

There are certain generalisations used in standard methods for predicting the distribution of fall-out deposited from the radioactive cloud of a nuclear explosion. The geology of the terrain where the bomb is dropped will affect the size of fall-out particles, so varying the distances over which these wind-borne particles are carried. Thus there will be different results for bombs burst on cities, over fields or over water.

The elliptical contours of the idealised fall-out patterns illustrated in Figure 3.4 assume perfectly uniform conditions, with a wind speed and direction remaining fixed over a large area and over a period of many hours or even days. The cross-wind dimensions of the theoretical ellipses represent an attempt to take into account the average effect of 'wind shear'—variations in wind direction at different altitudes—but this, too, is a simplification. In fact the total area affected by fall-out from a single large bomb may well extent to hundreds of thousands of square kilometres.

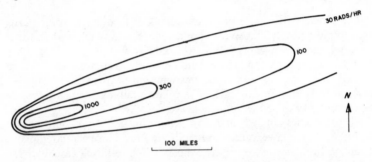

Figure 3.4. Idealised fall-out radiation dose rate contours for a 10 megaton, 50% fission ground-burst and an effective wind speed of 30 mph
Source: Glasstone and Dolan (1977) p.434 Fig. 9 100a

In reality local variations in weather conditions cause a much more complex pattern, as shown by the monitoring of fall-out from American weapons tests in the Pacific in the 1950s (Figure 3.5). Some of the radioactive material may be precipitated with rain or snow. There may be localised 'hot spots' formed where radiation levels are very high, compensated for by other less heavily affected areas. Once the fall-out particles have reached the ground, it is probable that some will be washed away by rain into sewers, rivers, reservoirs etc. or into the soil.

Some American computer models incorporate actual wind data, and can represent some of these complexities, but they are mostly used for research. They require sophisticated computing resources. The Working Party received no evidence of the use of such models in the British context. For military and civil defence planning purposes, there seems little point in trying to incorporate factors which are highly

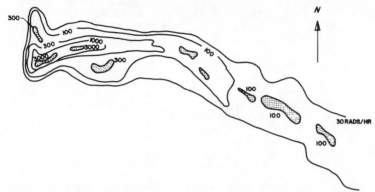

Figure 3.5. What actual dose rate contours might be like for the weapon of
Figure 3.4, as a result of variations in local meteorological and surface conditions.
The total area of contamination is about the same, but there are local 'hot spots'
(shown shaded)
Source: Glasstone and Dolan (1977) p.434 Fig. 9. 100b

changeable (and unpredictable). Instead the attempt is made, with the
idealised elliptical contours, to allow for *average* weather conditions, in
particular, prevailing wind directions and speeds. According to
Glasstone and Dolan (p.423): 'Although they [the idealised patterns]
will undoubtedly underestimate the fall-out in some locations and
overestimate it in others, the evaluation of the gross fall-out problem
over the whole area affected should not be greatly in error.'

Average wind conditions may nevertheless be subject to great
variations if taken month by month or on a seasonal basis; and these
variations can have significant consequences for casualty estimates.

Steadman and Openshaw have carried out some experiments with
their computer model, to investigate these effects for the UK. They
altered the assumed wind direction and wind speed in the 'Square Leg'
pattern of attack. (In the exercise itself the wind was taken to be
southerly at 24 km/hr.) They varied wind speeds between 12.8 and
40 km/hr, and looked at southerly, westerly and south-westerly wind
directions. The total casualties are, of course, dependent on many
factors; and the estimated fall-out casualties will vary with protective
factors and dose/injury models (as discussed below) as well as with the
meteorological conditions.

The figures in Table 3.12 give some indication of the possible order
of magnitude of changes due to wind effects. An average protective
factor of five is assumed throughout.

Table 3.12. Effects on total casualties (millions) from blast and fall-out, in the 'Square Leg' attack, of varying wind speed and direction (Openshaw and Steadman, 1983b)

	Wind speed	
Wind direction	12.8 km/hr	40 km/hr
Southerly	28.4	30.4
South-westerly	28.2	30.7
Westerly	30.4	33.8

With a higher wind speed the fall-out particles are spread in a given time (and hence at a given level of radioactivity) over a greater distance. The effects of wind direction are a complex function of whether population centres lie down-wind of ground-burst explosions in any given pattern of attack.

Protective factors of shelters (PF)

Any kind of shelter or enclosure will provide some protection against ionising radiation—principally gamma rays—from fall-out. The effectiveness depends on the materials, the thickness of the walls and roof, the overall geometrical form of the shelter, and its relationship to neighbouring structures. Fall-out particles tend to be deposited on horizontal surfaces—on the ground and on water, but also on flat or gently sloping roofs. Ideally, a shelter should be some distance from these surfaces. For example, the middle floors of a high-rise block are preferable as fall-out shelters, being further both from ground and roof. In a deep-plan building, such as an office block, it would be best to shelter in the centre of the lower floors. Immediately adjoining buildings can provide protection: a terraced house provides better shelter than a semi-detached or detached property. Worst of all in this respect is a bungalow.

The degree of protection offered in each case is measured as a *protective factor* or PF, which expresses the ratio of the dose received outside the shelter to that received inside. In a shelter with a PF of 5, therefore, the radiation dose received inside would be one fifth of that received in the open. Some values for the PFs of typical houses and other buildings in Britain are quoted by the Home Office in *Nuclear Weapons* (1974)[35] p.55 Table 23. These are reproduced in Table 3.13. It should be emphasised however that these values relate to buildings

Table 3.13. Approximate protective factors in ground floor refuge rooms of typical British housing with timber upper floors and with windows and external doors blocked (Home Office 1974)[35]

Types of housing	Protective factor
Bungalow	5–10
Detached two storey	15
Semi-detached two-storey 11 inch cavity walls	25–30
Semi-detached two-storey 13½ inch brick walls	40
Terraced two-storey	45
Terraced back-to-back	60
Blocks of flats and offices — lower floors	50–500
— Second floor and above (decreasing)	50–20

specially modified to serve as fall-out shelters. It is assumed that windows and external doorways have been blocked, and that a 'refuge room' has been constructed in the most advantageous position in the building. This room would be lined with dense materials — bags or boxes of sand, heavy furniture etc. — as in the instructions given in the *Protect and Survive*[32] leaflet. The calculated protective factor then relates to the interior of this refuge. Unadapted buildings would have much lower PFs than these. For instance an end-of-terrace house without openings blocked might have a PF of 10.

Protective factors of special-purpose fall-out shelters could also vary over a wide range. The Home Office describes several possible types in *Domestic Nuclear Shelters: Technical Guidance* (1981)[17]. Types 1a and 1b are improvised designs to be built in the garden at short notice, on a timber or scaffolding framework, with timber and earth cover. They are both calculated to have PFs greater than 40. Type 2 is a variant of the World War II 'Morrison' shelter consisting of a steel table surrounded with bricks, sand or other heavy materials. It is intended to be placed in the ground floor or basement of a house, and is strong enough to withstand the collapse of the house on top of it. The PF is greater than 70.

Type 3 is a pre-fabricated steel shelter similar to the World War II 'Anderson'. It is sunk in the ground and covered over with earth. The PF is 'not less than 200'. Type 4 is a permanent reinforced concrete below-ground shelter with a PF in excess of 300. A variety of commercial designs of permanent shelter have been on the market in Britain in the last two years. These are claimed by their manufacturers to have PFs in some cases as high as several thousand. Even vehicles would provide a little protection against radiation; for instance a car might have a PF of 1.5.

The methods of calculating protective factors are only approximate. The Home Office procedures, for example, assume that the building is a simple rectangle. Averages are used for the thicknesses of walls, floors and roofs. The assumption is made that no radioactive material is deposited on window-sills or other external projections from the walls, and that none enters the building.

Some of these approximations have been criticised (for example in the *London After the Bomb* study[31] Appendix 3 pp.108–12) as likely to lead to over-optimistic PF values. In practice, fall-out particles, just like other airborne debris, would very likely pile up on sills and in gutters, lodge in crevices, and enter the building through gaps. The averaging of wall thicknesses results in somewhat higher calculated PFs than if the thinner parts—the windows and doors—are considered separately.

More significant, however, are other factors that could affect the safety of the entire civilian population. First, there is the psychological question about whether, given the stresses of nuclear war, people could take effective sheltering precautions. At present the number of permanent below-ground fall-out shelters available to the general public in the UK is rather small. In a surprise attack it might not be possible even to reach those shelters.

If, during an international crisis, sufficient warning were given of a possible attack, people would have the time to prepare emergency shelters following Home Office recommendations. Doubts have been cast on the availability of sufficient supplies of suitable materials (bricks, plywood, scaffolding etc.). Some members of the population (the old, the disabled) might not be physically capable of the building work. Only a certain fraction of houses in cities have gardens suitable for outdoor shelters. Relatively few British houses have basements: in London, for example, only 3½ per cent of the population have access to a basement suitable for sheltering. People might have other priorities if nuclear attack seemed imminent—contacting relatives, or fleeing the cities and heading for the country.

Assuming people are successful in building and equipping refuges in advance of an attack, or before fall-out arrives, there is the further question of whether they will be able to stay inside for the whole danger period. The Home Office designs of expedient shelter are extremely cramped. The occupants would certainly be frightened and anxious, possibly seriously ill or injured. Conditions would be insanitary. Food and water might run out, and morale would deteriorate.

Arrangements exist for warning people, by radio or other means, about the extent of fall-out hazards, and for issuing the 'all-clear' signal (see Chapter 4). But these arrangements are not foolproof. Shocked people or people desperately seeking relatives or friends might ignore the warnings in any case. The required sheltering period is often taken to be two weeks, or longer depending on local fall-out conditions. It could vary in practice between a few days and more than a month. The protective factor of a shelter obviously applies for the occupants only so long as they remain inside. If people go out for appreciable lengths of time, so the average PF used in calculating the accumulated doses they receive must be reduced. (In normal everyday life a PF of about 3 would apply, allowing for the proportion of time people spend in and out of doors.) With high levels of radioactivity outside, dangerous or fatal effects could result from this exposure.

A second important factor relating to radiation protection is the effect of blast damage in reducing the effective PF. This could be serious and very extensive. Even blast damage to doors or tiled roofs, or the breaking of windows, could lower protective factors. At Hiroshima, houses generally suffered light damage out to 3½ km from ground zero, where the peak overpressure was about 1.5 psi. Windows were, however, broken at a radius of 15 km by overpressures of only a fraction of a pound per square inch — and in exceptional cases were broken as far as 27 km away.

In Openshaw and Steadman's study[33] of the 'Square Leg' attack, some 80,000 km², or roughly one third of the land area of the UK, was found to be subjected to overpressures of 1 psi or greater. Since these are principally the inhabited parts of Britain, it is plausible to suppose that the majority of windows in the country would be broken as a result. Windows could be blocked again, but this would require rapid action and suitable materials to hand. The *London After the Bomb* study group found that the 'Square Leg' bombs subjected 75 per cent of the GLC area to overpressures of at least 2 psi. As the same authors point out, the Home Office Type 1 designs of improvised garden shelter will only withstand peak overpressures of 1.5 psi. They would be demolished by blast in most of London before they could serve their intended function of providing fall-out protection. In zones more seriously affected by blast damage, little shelter of any kind against radiation would remain intact.

Various authors use a wide range of values for protective factors in making estimates of fall-out casualties. Rotblat in *Nuclear Radiation in Warfare* (1981)[3] recommends that a PF value of 5 be taken for acute effects of radiation, and 3 for longer-term effects.

The OTA do not offer their own calculations of fall-out casualties, but instead quote a variety of studies carried out for or by the US

Department of Defense, the US Arms Control and Disarmament Agency, and the American intelligence community. Values used for protective factors range very widely. At the low end, with no civil defence precautions taken at all, a PF of three is assumed for the entire population. In other studies, for those people in houses or buildings other than special purpose shelters, an average value of 5 or 6 is generally taken. Meanwhile for those with access to fall-out shelters proper, PF values of 10 to 40 or higher are assumed. According to the OTA, the numerical effect on predicted casualties of raising PF values much above 40 is fairly negligible.

In the Home Office computer model a 'spectrum' of PF values is used, rather than a single average, to correspond to the distribution of house types on a national basis. In the sample results given by Butler for an attack on military and city targets with 193 Mt (Table 3.6, Attack A) the protective factor spectrum is taken to represent 'general adherence to *Protect and Survive* advice . . . as regards fall-out precautions.' Butler does not specify the actual numerical values used, and the Home Office representative told the inquiry that the precise assumptions made here by Butler were unavailable. The assumed average level of PF value was however somewhat greater than 20. The resulting predicted number of fall-out deaths is less than one million.

The Home Office representative described a provisional estimate of the distribution of protective factors of current UK housing stock which has been issued for guidance to Scientific Advisers and is presently in use for casualty estimation. These figures have been derived by '. . . (a) selecting a range of representative house types for which estimates of the protective factors in the best location within the house (but without special adaptation) have been made, and (b) estimating (via liaison with Directorate of Works) the distribution of these types in the UK as a whole.' The values are as follows:

% of dwellings:	2	4	27	34	18	8	7
Protective factor	2	5	9	18	26	40	70

This gives an overall average PF of 21. The Home Office adds that these figures '. . . may well be modified when used in assessments, through assumptions about precautionary measures, regime followed, modified population distribution, etc.'

The results of all these variations in PF value on total casualties are very marked. For a series of American studies quoted by the OTA of a 'counterforce' attack on US ICBM silos, the calculated number of deaths, assuming there was no evacuation of the population, ranged between 2 and 22 million. The high figure relates approximately to a PF of 3 and the low to a PF of 25 or more. On the assumption that people who lived near to fall-out shelters presently existing in the US made use of those shelters, the total was calculated at 14 million deaths.

For the British situation, Openshaw and Steadman have made experiments with a series of different protective factors in the 'Square Leg' scenario (Table 3.7 Attack B). For average PFs of between 1 and 40 right across the country, the results are as follows:

Table 3.14. Effects on total casualties (millions) from blast and fall-out, in the 'Square Leg' attack, of varying protective factor assumptions. (Wind southerly, 24 km/hr) (Openshaw and Steadman 1983b)

Average nationwide PF:	1	4	10	20	40
All casualties (millions):	40.6	30.6	26.8	25.1	24

Casualties caused by blast alone amount to 23.6 million. Thus the additional casualties due to fall-out (burns injuries are not counted here) range from 0.4 million to 17 million. A striking feature of these calculations is how relatively insensitive the predicted numbers of fall-out casualties are to changes of PF value in the range 10 and above, by comparison with the extreme sensitivity in the range 1 to 10. These figures may be compared with the Home Office results reported in Table 3.6 (scenario A) for a similar weight and pattern of attack. The fact that the protective factor 'spectrum' used by Butler, with an average value in excess of 20, gives fewer than a million fall-out deaths, is broadly consistent with Openshaw and Steadman's results above.

On the question of the reduction of protective factors as a result of blast damage, the Home Office told the Working Party that no allowance for this effect is made in their current model: 'We recognise that a degradation effect would occur and that it would be desirable to allow for it. However, there is no reliable information available to us on which to base quantitative estimates, and moreover, it is believed that the effect is likely to be small, on the basis of observations of the behaviour of fall-out-like particles (e.g. volcanic dust).' These latter remarks can only be intended to apply nevertheless to cases of light or moderate damage. Clearly where houses are completely demolished, as in the A and B damage rings, the effective PF for survivors of blast must be 1.

The *London After the Bomb* group by contrast take explicit account, in calculating PFs, of the effects of blast (Appendix 3 pp.108–112). They take the four blast damage zones described by the OTA in calculating blast casualties, with peak overpressures of greater than 12, 5-12, 2-5 and 1-2 psi. For each of these zones they estimate the approximate area of apertures caused by the blast effects on a typical structure, compared with the total undamaged area of roof and walls. They assume that this can be related to the ratio of the radiation dose received from fall-out which has entered the building, to the open-air, unshielded dose. They make estimates separately for houses and for flats. From these they calculate average PFs for each blast damage zone. Because of uncertainties in the calculations they quote a range for the value in each case. The figures are conservative, nevertheless, in that they do *not* allow for any increase in the radiation dose from fall-out *outside* buildings received through the apertures.

The results for predicted casualties in the 'Square Leg' attack on London are illustrated in Table 3.15. Openshaw and Steadman have experimented with very similar blast-dependent ranges of PF values for

Table 3.15. Estimated protective factors for blast-damaged housing and resulting total casualties (blast plus fall-out, millions) in London and in the UK, for the 'Square Leg' attack. (Figures for London from *London After the Bomb*[31] Table 5 pp.38-9 and Table 8 p.111; for UK from Openshaw and Steadman (1983b)[33])

Blast damage zones	Typical damage	PF range (London) Lower limit	PF range (London) Upper limit	PF Range (UK) Low	PF Range (UK) Medium	PF Range (UK) High
More than 12 psi	Houses and flats completely destroyed	1	1	1	1	1
5-12 psi	Most housing destroyed, walls blown down, roofs removed	1	2	1	1	2
2-5 psi	Severe roof damage, walls cracked	2	5	1.5	2	5
1-2 psi	Windows smashed, doors blown in, some roof tiles removed	5	10	4	5	8
Less than 1 psi				5	8	10
Total casualties (Blast plus fall-out, millions):		London 5.8	5.3	UK 30.9	29.3	27.6

the 'Square Leg' attack over the whole country; their results are also shown in the table. In both cases the wind is southerly, at 24 km/hr.

The authors of *London After the Bomb* incline to the view that the lower limits of their specified ranges are the more realistic. The results given by Openshaw and Steadman for the whole UK in Table 3.7, both Attacks B and C, are calculated on the basis of their 'medium' range above. The effects on total casualties of the various ranges are appreciable though not so marked naturally as the effects of the very large changes in average nationwide PFs illustrated previously.

Radiation dose/injury relationships

In order to convert estimated radiation doses into numbers of predicted casualties, it is necessary to make some assumptions about the dose which will cause serious injury and death. It is conventional to express the effects of a given level of radiation dose in terms of the probability that a certain percentage of a large number of people exposed to that dose will die. A value often quoted is that dose which results in 50 per cent deaths and 50 per cent survivors, and which is referred to as the 'median lethal dose' or LD-50. Other dose levels will cause correspondingly lower or higher percentages of deaths, besides cases of radiation sickness of varying severity.

It is important to specify what precisely is referred to by an LD-50 figure. Values are generally taken to refer to healthy adults (LD-50s would be lower for sick people, and also for children because of their smaller body size), and to acute exposures of the whole body, not separate limbs. By 'acute' is meant generally exposures over one day or less, but sometimes the term applies to exposures over an hour or two only.

The dose may be measured at the surface tissues, at 'mid-line' tissues, or to the bone marrow. LD-50 values for surface tissue doses will be higher (by about one third) than doses to bone marrow, because the flesh attenuates the radiation reaching the bones. Values for the LD-50 may also either assume that those exposed receive hospital treatment, or that they do not. The units of measurement may be either rads or roentgens. Their value, however, is fairly close. For the gamma rays likely to be produced from nuclear weapons, and for doses measured in air, one R (roentgen) = 0.87 rad. For doses measured in soft tissue, one R = 0.96 rad. Another unit in use is the Gray; it is equal to 100 rads (see Introduction).

As for the actual numerical value which the LD-50 should take, this is a subject where many doubts and difficulties exist. A recent report from the British Institute of Radiology, 'The Radiological Effects of Nuclear War'[38], describes the situation:

There have been fewer than 100 documented instances of significant human whole-body exposure in peacetime and neither in these cases nor in the wartime attacks on Japan was the dosage known at all accurately. Several of the accident cases received massive doses of the order of tens of Grays and thus convey little information about the level of the mean lethal dose in man. In the accident cases also, intensive therapy designed to modify the clinical course of the radiation damage was usually available, while in Japan many of the irradiated patients had other injuries as well and died without any permanent record of the clinical signs and symptoms of radiation reaction. Estimates of the mean lethal dose for an irradiated human population without access to intensive therapy are therefore uncertain.

As long ago as 1949 the figure of 450 roentgens (measured in air) was chosen as the median of a number of educated guesses for the human LD-50/60 which is shorthand for 'the dose at which 50% of the irradiated population would die within 60 days'. The corresponding absorbed dose at the mid-line of the adult body would be about 3.2 Gy. Some subsequent studies of the available data have suggested a somewhat lower figure. However, the curve of mortality versus dose is very steep at these high dose levels and it may be rather more accurate and equally relevant to the present discussion to consider the exposure which would lead to 90% mortality. It is claimed that this may lie between 500 and 600 roentgens (measured in air), corresponding to a mid-line dose of less than 4.3 Gy in an adult, or a surface dose of about 6 Gy. No person is known to have survived an evenly distributed torso or whole-body dose greater than 4.6 Gy mid-line (650 R in air) without medical treatment.

Professor P. J. Lindop of the Department of Radiobiology at St. Bartholomew's Hospital gave evidence to the Working Party on the LD-50 value in humans. She cited recent reports of the National Radiological Projection Board (NRPB-R52, November 1976 and NRPB-R87, July 1979) to the effect that the LD-50 is about 300 rads to the bone marrow, or about 400 rem surface dose (Figure 3.6). Professor Lindop comments: '. . . what is important in this dose-response curve is the steepness of the line. Within a 200 rad range the probability of death goes up from 2% to 85%, and it is reasonable to assume that the error on the measurement of dose would cover this range.' These values relate to healthy adults who do not receive treatment.

The prospect of improved short-term survival would be increased by treatment in a sterile unit in hospital with antibiotics, blood and fluid transfusions and in some cases bone marrow transplantation. The British Institute of Radiology (BIR) Report indicates that with good conventional medical treatment the LD-50 could be increased to over 5 Gy. The opportunities for such treatment in the conditions

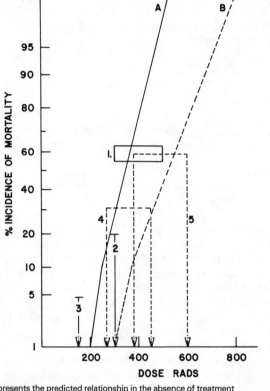

Curve A represents the predicted relationship in the absence of treatment

1   159 Hiroshima victims
2   22 Ewing's sarcoma patients   } No treatment
3   64 Marshall islanders

Curve B represents the predicted effect of treatment

4   8 Accident cases treated with antibiotics   } Simple support
5   6 Accident cases treated with bone marrow transplants } ie, antibiotic, blood
                                                               transfusion

Error bars for % mortality represent 95% confidence limits; dose shown where appropriate.

Figure 3.6. Dose-response curves for bone marrow deaths
Source: National Radiological Protection Board (1979)

following a large-scale nuclear attack would be extremely limited, or absent, in the devastated area.

As for American studies of nuclear radiation in warfare, Glasstone and Dolan (1977)[2] quote values, for doses to surface tissues received in one day or less, of an incidence of death between 0 per cent and 90 per cent in the range 200 to 600 rads. The Office of Technology Assessment[29] give figures for doses received in up to six or seven days of 450 rem for the LD-50, and 600 rem for 90 per cent mortality.

When a dose is divided or protracted over a longer period, it will tend to be less damaging than a similar single dose. The BIR Report indicates that the LD-50 for a dose protracted over one month would be 6 Gy compared with 4.5 Gy for one week.

Many of the injured in a nuclear attack would suffer some combination of mechanical injuries, burns and radiation. As the BIR Report says:

A radiation dose well below the lethal level could make recovery from the other injuries more difficult. Wound healing is inhibited in irradiated animals and the immune defences against infection are reduced. Serious burns cause shock and fluid loss and combined burn and radiation injuries have been shown to be synergistic, that is, to lead to greater mortality than the simple addition of the casualties to be expected from each of the separate insults.

The study by the *London After the Bomb*[31] group illustrated in Table 3.5 makes assumptions broadly in accordance with the values cited above. The authors base their figures on data published by the National Radiological Protection Board (NRPB-R87, 1979 pp.43-4). They choose an LD-50 value (surface tissues) of 400 rads for doses accumulated up to two weeks, for those who do not suffer injuries from other causes. They justify this value on the grounds that hospital treatment cannot be expected to be available; that the greater part (perhaps 80 per cent) of the two-week dose is received in the first two days after an attack; that the total dose will also continue to accumulate after the two-week period; and that LD-50s for children and the elderly would be lower than for the average adult. For those who are counted as injured also by burns or blast effects, the authors take an LD-50 of 300 rads, to allow for synergism.

Until fairly recently the Home Office took an LD-50 of 450 (rads or roentgens; surface tissues; acute doses) for use in casualty estimation. In 1975, however, the Scientific Advisory Branch sought new advice on this subject from the Protection Against Ionising Radiation Committee (PIRC) of the Medical Research Council. A working party was set up under the Chairmanship of Dr J. C. Vennart and reported in the form of a letter to the Home Office in 1977. A number of supporting scientific papers, including papers by Dr Vennart and Dr R. H. Mole, were also submitted. These have not yet been published.

The Home Office asked the PIRC working party:

What is the present best estimate of the immediate biological effects on man of brief exposures to gamma radiation? (By brief we mean exposures received within a few minutes and by immediate we mean effects becoming evident to the affected individual within three months of a brief exposure.) It would be helpful if such information could be set out in a dose/effects table.

The PIRC replied:

Over the last 26 years the value of the brief exposure to energetic gamma radiation which would cause half those receiving it to die within the next 2-3 months, that is, the LD-50, has been stated to be 450 R . . . A review of the available information suggests that this is an underestimate but also that there is a lack of appropriate observations in man to allow a statement of the value applicable without qualifications to a normal population consisting very largely of ordinary fit persons. All accident cases involving extensive damage to other tissues or receiving treatment by extraordinary measures had perforce to be put on one side since the question requires an answer relating to more-or-less uniform gamma radiation and applying to circumstances in which hospital treatment is not available.

The PIRC supported its estimates of an LD-50 value with evidence from some 20 patients receiving radiation therapy and some 19 victims of accidents. Most of these received doses in the range 150 to 350 rads, and none received doses in excess of 370 rads. Only one person in the sample died. Extrapolating from this basis, the PIRC proposed for generally fit persons briefly exposed an LD-50 of 450 rads mean bone marrow dose. (This would correspond to a surface tissue dose of about 600 rads.) 'The uncertainty of extrapolation,' they say, 'is such that the LD-50 may be in the range 400–500 rad mean bone marrow dose.' The dose level they take to kill almost everyone is 600 rad bone marrow dose (about 800 rad to surface tissues). The resulting deaths would almost all occur within 60 days after exposure.

The PIRC added in commentary:

There will always be a small proportion of individuals in a normal population who, because they are severely ill or dying from natural causes, will be more susceptible to death after a given exposure to radiation than the normally fit, and they have been disregarded . . . . Helpful treatment for whole-body irradiation under emergency conditions is hardly possible . . . . There is no simple means of preventing infection during the weeks after a brief whole-body exposure and treatment of a recognised infection when it occurs is of uncertain value.

Table 3.16 was supplied by the PIRC to the Home Office for use in casualty estimation, with the caveat that it is provided 'as a working hypothesis only and must be regarded as only tenuously based on evidence.' It has been incorporated into the current version of the Home Office computer model, as described by Bentley (1981)[34] p.18, in the form of the assumed relationships of death and serious injury to dose level illustrated in Figure 3.7 (note that the scale for dose values refers to rads-in-air, not bone marrow doses, and related to the Operational Evaluation Dose (OED) value—see below).

Table 3.16. Dose from energetic gamma rays and level of effect (PIRC Working Party advice to Home Office Scientific Advisory Branch, 1977)

Mean marrow dose for brief exposure (rads)	Expected mortality* %	Expected second phase of incapacitation in 4th-6th weeks	
		Symptoms	Effect on blood count
600	95+	severe in 100%	marked
450	about 50	severe in 100%	marked
300	0-5	severe in 50%	marked
200	0	none	moderate
100	0	none	slight

*The upper two levels of this table are based on judgements, not on observations.

These values relate, however, to doses received within a few minutes. Where doses are received in periods of hours or days, they are modified, in casualty calculation by hand or in the computer model, in accordance with what the Home Office terms the 'Operational Evaluation Dose' or OED formula. This allows for two successive mechanisms of recovery, one short-term and the other longer-term, as the Home Office explains in the second of their questions addressed to the PIRC:

Arising out of reports of studies carried out at the MRC Radiobiology Unit the Home Office has adopted a 'radiological recovery formula' which allows for a recovery by the human body from a dose of 150 rads received within a short time plus a capability of recovery at a rate of 10 rads per day from subsequent doses. As a result of the applications of this formula, the policy has been adopted that an *Operational Equivalent Dose* can be calculated by noting the dose registered on the dose meter and subtracting from this 150 plus 10 each day subsequent to the commencement of the exposure. The question then is: Is this Operational Equivalent Dose to be regarded as the acute dose equivalent of the dose accumulated in time?

The PIRC replied:

For the purpose of assessing the likelihood of death caused by protracted radiation exposure . . . OED can be regarded as the equivalent of the brief acute exposure of the same numerical value. The same formula can be used whether exposure is more-or-less uniformly protracted or is intermittent, regardless of hourly dose-rate. The formula does not necessarily restrict an allowable exposure to 10 units per day but the exposure received in any given 24 hours should not be planned to exceed say 20 units or so. Direct experiment in laboratory mice has shown that there is no particular biological significance in an exposure with dose rate decreasing as in a fall-out field. The OED formula applies to lethality, not to delayed effects. A negative value has no meaning.

The PIRC explain that the word 'unit' here refers to the quantity to be chosen as appropriate for civil defence dose meters. All dose values in their advice to the Home Office are given in terms of mean marrow dose, as in the table above.

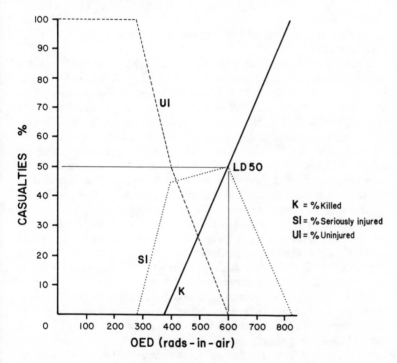

Figure 3.7. Radiation dose casualty assumptions used in the current version of the Home Office computer model. 'OED' refers to the value of the 'operational evaluation dose' formula

Source: Bentley (1981) p.18 Fig.15.

The effect of using the OED formula is thus to raise the effective LD-50 value for exposures received over periods of more than a few minutes. As indicated in the question and answer above, the OED formula previously took the form:

$$OED = x - 150 - 10t \text{ rads}$$

where x is the actual dose received and t is the number of days after the start of exposure. In the most recent version of the Home Office computer model, this expression has been altered, however (Bentley 1981[34], p.17), to:

$$OED = x - 200 - 15t \text{ rads}$$

(Although this version of the formula does not appear in the PIRC advice of 1977.)

Thus for doses received over periods of between several hours and one day, the model incorporates an effective LD-50 value of 600 rads (bone marrow) equivalent to a surface tissue dose of 800 rads. For doses received over longer periods, an additional 15 rads is added for every day of exposure. The Home Office representative told the Working Party that in the model, the value for the OED for each exposed group in the population is calculated to the end of seven days. Thus the effective LD-50 value taken for this period would be just over 900 rads surface tissue dose. Higher and lower levels of dose than the median lethal value would be modified by the use of the OED formula in a similar way, as Bentley's Figure 3.7 illustrates.

We leave for debate amongst radiobiologists the scientific merits of the various assumptions and arguments reviewed here, and would merely point to the very large difference between this effective LD-50 in the current Home Office model of more than 900 rads, and the figure previously quoted, for example by the British Institute of Radiology, of 450 rads, both applying to surface tissue doses received over one week. Professor Lindop in evidence to the inquiry was nevertheless critical specifically of the OED expression in its earlier form. She said '. . . from limited clinical experience and animal data I would expect that this dose rate [10 R per day] given after an acute dose of 150 R would result in severe bone marrow damage several weeks later. No data show that 10 R or more per day can be repaired indefinitely.'

Openshaw and Steadman's computer model makes use of a modified version of Bentley's assumptions, in which the dose/effects relationships illustrated in Figure 3.7 are applied to the actual dose received (and not the value given by the OED formula). This implies an LD-50 of 450 rads, taken in their case for accumulated doses measured over 14 days. The figures for fall-out casualties in Table 3.7 are calculated on the basis. In both the Steadman and Openshaw and the Home Office models those who are seriously injured simultaneously from radiation and other effects are assumed to die.

Openshaw and Steadman have experimented using their model on the 'Square Leg' scenario, with their own radiation dose assumptions as against the assumptions which Bentley makes in the Home Office model incorporating the revised OED formula. Total predicted casualties (blast plus fall-out) in the first case are 34 million, in the second case 28.5 million, assuming a 24 km/hr wind and a national average protective factor of five. For a PF of ten, the corresponding values are 30 million and 26.5 million. Where average PF values are taken to be much higher than this, as for example in the Home Office results reported in Table 3.6, the difference in absolute numbers of casualties predicted on the two sets of assumptions would be less marked.

Implications of uncertainties and discrepancies in assumptions for predicted casualties on a national scale

In concluding our discussion of these various estimates of casualties, we should reiterate the caveats with which we began. All the figures quoted so far refer only to the short-term effects of a nuclear attack: to those who would be killed and injured, or else 'sentenced to death' from radiation sickness, in the first few days or weeks following an attack. Many causes of death and injury which would undoubtedly occur have not been taken into account because of the difficulty or impossibility of calculation: fires, food and water shortage, epidemics, lack of health care, lack of shelter and heating, and the possible breakdown of law and order. Some of these are discussed in the following section, as are the longer-term consequences of radiation exposure, and the possibility of certain complex environmental and ecological effects. Other factors which are in principle calculable but have nevertheless also been omitted are the possibility of fall-out reaching Britain from the Continent, and the special fall-out hazards created if nuclear power stations or reprocessing and storage facilities for nuclear materials were successfully attacked. For these reasons, despite all the uncertainties of calculation discussed, most of the total figures given in Tables 3.3–3.7 can be expected to err on the side of underestimating casualties.

We have throughout this chapter contrasted the calculation methods used variously by the Home Office, by American authorities and by British studies (specifically those made by members of the organisation Scientists Against Nuclear Arms). We would re-emphasise that the methods and figures used in these latter studies are themselves drawn almost exclusively from American government and military sources— the Office of Technology Assessment study, the US Department of Defense, and Glasstone and Dolan's book—and that these authorities can be expected to be, if anything, conservative in their assumptions.

Of the various discrepancies discussed, it may be asked which are the more significant for total casualties in, say, a 200 Mt level of attack on the UK? In roughly descending order of importance they would appear to be:

(1) Blast casualty rates

We have seen how in Butler's Attack A (Table 3.6) the use of assumptions similar to those of the OTA raises predicted blast deaths to 27 million, from a figure of 16 million for the current Home Office assumptions.

(2) Differences in protective factor assumptions and the linkage of protective factor values to levels of blast damage

We have seen how predicted fall-out deaths vary between less than one million for Butler's Attack A with PF values equivalent to a national average of over 20 (and no linkage to blast effects), and 11 million in Openshaw and Steadman's Attack B for a national average PF of 8, reduced from this value in areas suffering significant blast damage.

(3) Differences in LD-50 values for radiation doses

We have seen how the use of a simple LD-50 value of 450 rads with no allowance for possible short-term repair mechanisms has the effect of adding some four or five million casualties from fall-out (assuming average PFs between 5 and 10, wind speed 24 km/hr) to the totals given by the Home Office LD-50 value of 600 rads together with their use of the OED formula.

(4) The inclusion or omission of burns caused by direct thermal radiation

We have seen how this might have the effect of adding two or three million deaths if five per cent of the population were exposed, by contrast with the Home Office assumption of none exposed and no burns casualties.

Calculations by Openshaw and Steadman (1983a)[20] indicate that the combined effects of all the differences between their own and the Home Office's computer model is for the former to predict roughly twice or even two and a half times the total number of casualties, for an identical pattern and weight of attack.

A final very important cause of differences in national casualty estimates has nothing to do with assumptions relating to weapons effects or casualty rates, nor with the structure of the computer models used. It has to do with the issue raised at several points in the discussion above of the average yield of weapons assumed in an attack. It will be seen from Table 3.7 that Attack C results in 38.6 million deaths and 4.3 million injured, while Attack B ('Square Leg') results in 26.7 million deaths and 6.8 million injured. This is despite the fact that the total yield employed in Attack C is only some 25 Mt greater; *and* that Attack C is directed almost exclusively at military and strategic targets and does not, like 'Square Leg', include cities as targets in their own right.

The explanation lies in the numbers and average yields of weapons employed in either case: 125 warheads of average yield 1.57 Mt in Attack B, 340 warheads of average yield 0.65 Mt in Attack C. It is, unfortunately, those in Attack C which correspond to the types of Soviet weapons which are thought to be currently targeted on Britain, as discussed in Chapter 2. The consequence of an attack of this nature is for relatively high levels of blast overpressure to extend over most of the inhabited parts of the country, since military targets in Britain are, for the most part, either within or close to centres of population. This in turn results in lowered protective factors for houses in many areas. A significant proportion of the warheads targeted on hardened military installations and airfields are assumed to be ground-bursts. In these conditions the numbers of fall-out casualties are especially high. The argument which is sometimes advanced, that a 'counterforce' attack with low-yield weapons would be less damaging and produce fewer casualties, would thus seem at least for Britain to be the reverse of the truth.

Finally, we recall that in Chapter 2 we quoted several authorities, both in and out of Government, who took the view that attacks on the UK might well be made with total yields much greater than 200 megatons—perhaps even three or four times this quantity.

CHAPTER 4

The long-term medical effects
of nuclear explosions

*Following on from the immediate medical effects of a nuclear attack,
this chapter looks at the long-term medical effects on survivors of an
'average' attack for a period of about two years, paying special
attention to the problems likely to be experienced with shelter and
with water, food and power supplies. Account is taken, however, of
the much longer period over which the consequences of radiation
might be expected to continue. The long-term medical effects are of
less immediate significance than the basic needs of survivors for
water, food, shelter and power.*

Examination of the long-term effects of nuclear explosions implies
survival of the short-term effects detailed in Chapter 3. The notion that
rescue services could spring into action immediately after a nuclear
attack, in the same way that Civil Defence operated during the bombing
of cities in the last war, is dangerously unrealistic. By the time the
radiation hazard had fallen to acceptable levels for rescue attempts (and
this could take 14–21 days), most of the seriously injured would have
perished from haemorrhage, secondary infection or radiation sickness
compounded by dehydration, exposure and shock.

Environmental health

Water

Before anything else survivors of a nuclear explosion would need
adequate supplies of uncontaminated water. The most seriously injured
would be in greatest need of fluid replacement and would be the first to
die if this could not be administered. At best, small emergency supplies
in shelters or buildings left standing might be expected to meet the
basic needs of uninjured survivors for the first few days. Water is

necessary not only as part of the preparation of food but with fuel as part of the cooking process used to sterilise food.

We understand from an authority on water supplies that in peacetime the tankers available in the UK could carry and distribute water for essential purposes to just two per cent of the population. However, radiation levels immediately following a nuclear attack would prevent the distribution of any water at all unless there were suitably equipped emergency rescue squads available with adequate protective clothing.

Gamma radiation does not affect the purity of water. Contamination following a nuclear explosion is due to fall-out of radioactive isotopes in a fission or in a fission-fusion-fission reaction detonation. There are about 200 varieties of these isotopes, each with its own specific rate of spontaneous decay, measured in terms of its half life, which may vary from a fraction of a second to thousands of years. This is the reason why the radioactivity of fall-out decreases rapidly at first as the short-lived isotopes decay.

Covered water protected from fall-out would provide a safe supply so far as radiation is concerned, but main services would be destroyed and it might be impossible to restore even a limited service in the short term due to the likely shortages of skilled staff and materials. The majority of the UK's water supplies require pumping and this presumably would be impossible in many areas due to disrupted supplies.

Radioactive nuclide material in the fall-out is relatively insoluble in water and falls to the bottom of open containers, reservoirs and rivers. For this reason running streams are likely to be safe sources of water as long as the bed remains undisturbed. Despite this, if water is taken from ponds or reservoirs the surface layer should not be used in the early days after an attack.

It is claimed that rain always falls within a few hours of nuclear explosions, although the scientific explanation of this is unknown. If it does rain, large quantities of fall-out could be washed into sewers, streams, rivers or reservoirs, contaminating water which might otherwise have remained safe. Much of the surface fall-out would be washed into the soil.

Food

Like many other countries, the UK is served by a food distribution system which relies heavily on a complicated, energy-dependent transport network. Furthermore, despite a recent trend to move into the interior, food-processing plants, such as the two major flour mills in Tilbury and in Seaforth near Liverpool, are concentrated near seaports.

The food distribution system is likely to be extensively disrupted over much of the UK following a nuclear attack.

In the immediate aftermath of an attack, survivors would be able to live off tinned food if supplies could be salvaged from shops and supermarkets. However, Government contingency plans note that during the pre-attack period there would be increased demand for food and that this would result in shortages in the supply chain. It is suggested by Government that it might be necessary to control food supplies. Even then, 'No arrangements could ensure that every surviving household would have . . . 14 days' supply of food.'

The Government appears to base its plans on the reasonable assumption that there would be no significant food imports following a nuclear attack, and that peacetime food processing and distribution systems would cease to function. These plans, therefore, include the identification of major stocks of basic commodities and the notification of authorities as to the whereabouts of these stocks. There are also plans to disperse stocks normally held in areas liable to attack. There would be a transition from normal trading to Government control as the situation deteriorated.

In theory, the Government would quickly be able to make available Ministry of Agriculture, Fisheries and Food strategic stockpiles of reserves such as flour, sugar, refined fat, yeast and special biscuits. They note that these reserves do not constitute a balanced diet nor are they in quantities to 'meet needs of the population over a particular period'. The Working Party understands that the strategic stockpiles may contain only sufficient supplies to sustain a peacetime UK population for a few weeks. Both the population and the food reserves would suffer severe attrition in a nuclear attack and while the whereabouts of these stockpiles are not known, it is understood that some are near major cities while others are located in the countryside. Blast from explosions, particularly where food storage depots are sited within a radius of 10 to 20 kilometres of an area vulnerable to attack, may be sufficient to expose the food contents to radioactive fall-out. Damage to power supplies could cause great losses in frozen food in areas remote from the site of attack, unless it could be distributed and consumed before it deteriorated. Disruption of ports and the transport system would make the replacement of reserves improbable, or impossible, even if other countries were willing to send supplies.

Agriculture: the production of food

The UK has approximately 24 million hectares of land, of which 19 million hectares are given over to agriculture. It is estimated that in 1981 this country produced 85 per cent of its total meat supply and 96 per cent of its total cereal supply. However, these figures take no account of the import and export market nor, in the case of cereals, do they take account of the amount of cereal consumed by livestock.

Cereal production is concentrated in the eastern part of the country, while the bulk of livestock farming is in the west. Cereals are grown for animal feed as well as for human dietary needs and there are small stocks of cereals not normally considered fit for human consumption dispersed throughout the country. Approximately five-sixths of the nutritional value of a cereal is lost by feeding it to livestock, which need time and energy resources in order to develop to optimum weight for slaughter. In view of this, and the fact that livestock are more sensitive than plants to the effects of radiation, it might be worth slaughtering a number of animals and salting down the meat in the days after a nuclear attack. However, the majority of the UK salt supply comes from the Cheshire area and this would present major problems to do with organisation, communication and transport.

The main cereals grown in the UK are wheat, barley, oats, maize, rye and oilseed rape. UK wheat is normally used in the production of soft flour for biscuits and cakes and for pig and poultry feed. Barley is used for beer and whisky production and also for animal feed. Oats is used for animal feed and porridge. Maize in the UK is grown for the stem, leaf and half-grown pod. Rye is no longer produced on a large scale in the UK. Pulses such as peas and beans are grown for animal feed and for canning, drying and freezing. All these vegetables (except oilseed rape which contains a poison) may be consumed by humans; however, the fact that water is needed to render cereals edible and, to a lesser extent, that power processes are required to break down cereal to a form which is readily digestible by humans, would create difficulties.

We believe that survivors would be able to obtain enough food only by changing their dietary pattern to include a much greater amount of diverse cereals and vegetables than usual. Despite the difficulties of distribution, these foods would be more readily available and solve more nutritional problems than animal products. Of course, it would not be possible for members of the population with special dietary requirements to find appropriate foods.

Palatability of cereals would be a major problem. Experience in dealing with famine shows that there is difficulty in persuading people to eat sufficient quantities of cereal to obtain sufficient protein and energy. In Ghana, for example, attempts have been made to replace one type of sorghum with another, higher-yield variety. However, the population would not accept the new cereal, despite the higher yield, because of the unfamiliar flavour.

Farm animals are sensitive to the effects of radiation. For sheep the LD-50 is around 3.5 Gy and for cattle 4.4 Gy. In addition to external exposure by gamma rays, beta radiation is likely to contribute to the mortality of animals kept in the open. As well as burns to the skin, grazing beasts are likely to suffer from mucosal burns caused by internal radiation from the consumption of contaminated grass. It has been shown that the LD-50 is lowered markedly by combined internal and external radiation. Insects and vermin are much more resistant to radiation and it has been suggested that in the post-attack phase these might become a major public health problem, with a proliferation of flies and cockroaches and rats, for instance, contributing to the spread of disease.

There is a wide range of sensitivity to radiation amongst plants of various species differing by a factor of 500. It is likely that external beta radiation will also be important in crop damage, particularly for crops in the early growth stages when they are small and have only minimal protective tissues around the more sensitive growing regions. Because of the practical difficulties in studying the effects of beta radiation, most work on plants has been concerned with the effects of gamma radiation. The most sensitive crops, such as peas, have an LD-50 value of around 10 Gy but less vulnerable crops such as rice have an LD-50 of over 100 Gy. Grasses are more radiation-resistant and a dose of perhaps 200 Gy is needed to destroy grassland. Conifers are much more sensitive to radiation than deciduous trees.

The incorporation of radioactivity into food chains could have important medium- and long-term effects on the animal and human survivors. The main hazards from early fall-out are iodine 131 and other fission products which may cause extensive contamination of milk. Drinking fresh milk following a nuclear attack could cause high doses of radiation to the thyroid gland in particular; children are particularly vulnerable. To overcome this, it has been suggested that sodium iodide tablets should be made available to survivors in order to block the uptake of radioactive iodine into the thyroid gland. The distribution of this medicine, a 'simple' operation before a nuclear war, would probably be impossible to achieve afterwards.

After about a year strontium 90 (^{90}Sr) and caesium 137 (^{137}Cs) will be the most important nuclides remaining on the diet after the decay of the shorter-lived nuclides. During the first three years or so after a major nuclear exchange these harmful nuclides will mostly find their way into the diet as a result of global fall-out settling on vegetation.

After about three years the uptake of radionuclides through the root systems will begin to be of greater importance. Body burdens of strontium 90 and caesium 136 in people surviving for this length of time would depend on many variables including the type of diet consumed. A high milk diet would tend to lead to strontium 90 accumulation and caesium 137 would be especially noticeable in people eating a preponderance of meat. As far as is practicable, survivors would need to use processed milk products, such as hard cheeses, in which the radioactive mineral content is greatly reduced. Caesium 137 has a more rapid turnover than strontium 90 and its biological half life is only a few months, whereas strontium 90 is deposited mainly in bone and therefore has a much longer turnover time. Other factors which affect concentrations of radionuclides in the body include soil characteristics. For example, acidic soils lead to much higher levels of caesium 137 accumulating in milk or meat.

It has been suggested (Clayton, 1978)[16] that in a nuclear attack of 200 megatons, four-fifths of the land area of the UK, including nearly all farming areas, would experience little physical damage other than minor effects from direct blast and heat. This, however, is strongly contested by other commentators, including Steadman and the Swedish Royal Academy of Sciences journal *Ambio*[14], whose conclusions are discussed in Chapter 2. As transport and food processing systems will be disrupted, the survivors will have to use locally available food resources. It has been suggested (Jackson, 1979)[40] that a calorie intake of 2000 Kcal/head/day averaged over men, women and children is a reasonable basis on which to estimate what food resources would be required for survivors following an attack, many of whom would be doing hard manual work.

The effects of changes in atmospheric ozone concentrations

Whatever the level of damage by blast and radiation, the possibility of producing adequate quantities of food for the survivors of a nuclear attack would depend heavily on the climate in the following years. This in turn would be governed as much by atmospheric factors as by conditions prevailing on the ground.

In North America and the USSR, vast forests are found close to important urban strategic centres, so it may be expected that many wild uncontrolled fires would be started during a nuclear exchange. As a rough estimate, we might expect an input of 15–30 Teragrams (Tg) of nitrogen into the atmosphere as a result of forest fires. Such an emission of nitric oxides (NO_X) would be larger than that produced by the fireballs of the weapons themselves and would be comparable to the entire annual output of NO_X by industrial processes. Considering the critical role of NO_X in the production of tropospheric ozone, it is conceivable that there might be a large accumulation of ozone in the troposphere, leading to global photochemical smog conditions. More serious atmospheric consequences are likely to arise from fires started by the destruction of gas and oil wells. There are an estimated 600,000 such wells throughout the world, many of them concentrated in small areas likely to become prime targets in the event of a nuclear war. Much of the gas and oil released as a result of a nuclear attack would burn; this conflagration would typically add 20 Tg of nitrogen to the NO_X emitted by forest fires.

The effects of ozone on plant growth have been studied for several decades. The implications for agricultural crops may be particularly severe. A major Environmental Protection Agency (EPA)[41] report listed several types of decreases in crops yields. For instance:

A 30% reduction in the yield of wheat occurred when wheat at antheses (blooming) was exposed to ozone at 200 parts per billion volume (ppbv), four hours a day for seven days. Chronic exposures to ozone at 50-150 ppbv for 4-6 hours a day reduced yield in soya beans and corn grown under field conditions. The threshold for measurable effects for ozone appear between 50 and 100 ppbv for sensitive plant species . . . and this level of exposure can significantly inhibit plant growth and yields in certain species.

A major nuclear exchange in the northern hemisphere might produce an increase of average ground level ozone concentration of 160 ppbv with higher values to be expected in the wake of a mixture of forest fires and gas and oil well fires. It follows, therefore, that agricultural crops may be subjected to severe photochemical pollutant stress.

The atmospheric effects of the many forest fires started by a nuclear war would be severe. It appears highly unlikely that agricultural crop yields would be sufficient to feed more than a small part of the remaining population, so many of the survivors of the initial effects of the nuclear war could die of starvation in the immediate first post-war years.

The impact would be different if a nuclear attack started in the winter months. The forest areas lost to fire might be only half as large and photochemical reactions would be slower due to reduced solar radiation and lower temperatures during the northern winter. However, because of the low winter sun, the obscurity caused by smoke would be greater.

Oxides of nitrogen (NO_X) promote ozone formation in the troposphere. In the stratosphere, where the chemical composition and light spectrum are quite different, the effect of NO_X is to catalyse ozone destruction. Whereas ozone is an undesirable pollutant in the troposphere, in the stratosphere it performs the important function of shielding the Earth's surface from biologically damaging ultraviolet radiation. Reduction of the ozone concentration would cause a cooling of the stratosphere. By absorbing ultraviolet sunlight, ozone heats the atmosphere at this level and causes the temperature inversion that is responsible for the high degree of resistance to vertical mixing. In the stratosphere NO_2 is the major component of the nitric oxides (NO_X). The absorption of solar radiation by the NO_2 heats the stratosphere. The net effect at mid-latitudes in the perturbed stratosphere is heating below about 22 kilometres and cooling above.

The long-term prospects for agriculture

The first harvest following a nuclear attack would present a host of problems. Even if the attack were to take place immediately following a previous main harvest or in the late growing season, the large amount of power needed to dry grain to a moisture content of less than 20 per cent for storage is unlikely to be available. Modern methods of harvesting, using combine harvesters, also depend upon adequate fuel supplies.

Meanwhile, it is unrealistic to assume that survivors would be able to switch to traditional methods of agriculture. Even if a sufficient number of old-fashioned implements, such as scythes, were available, the techniques of using them have been lost. With mechanisation, the labour force in agriculture (which once claimed up to 30 per cent of the nation's manpower) has dwindled to 3 per cent.

The next major hurdle would be planting a new crop. Many modern seed hybrids are not self-seeding. Current methods of cultivation rely particularly on nitrogen fertilizers, most of which are produced by ICI on Teesside—a region vulnerable to nuclear attack. Herbicides are also important in cultivation, although these may be held in stockpiles on farms as they are used in much smaller quantities than fertilizers. However, planting and the subsequent care of crops depend on the use of machinery such as tractors and crop-sprayers which, once again, would be a drain on remaining reserves of fuel.

According to Government plans as set out in ES/1/79, regional centres of government would assume the overall direction of food supplies following a nuclear attack. The plans provide for each centre to have a regional food officer and a regional agricultural officer with, below them, a series of divisional food and agricultural officers. Local authorities would appoint county and district food officers to assume responsibility for food distribution and conservation in their respective territories. Some provision is made for a post-attack communications system to encompass food officers. According to ES/1/79:

Plans for the control of agriculture are based on groupings of agricultural holdings. As a national average, each group would comprise about 800 agricultural holdings controlled by an agricultural officer normally having two assistant agricultural officers reporting to him. The agricultural officer would receive general instructions regarding policy and supplies from the divisional office. The link between assistant agricultural officers and farmers will be from wardens appointed by the Ministry of Agriculture, Fisheries and Food on the basis of one for each 20 or so farms depending on the topography of the area and size and type of the individual holdings.

Help from foreign powers may be available following a nuclear attack. However, this can not be relied on, and it might take some months or even years for any substantial assistance to reach survivors.

Fuel

Our discussions of water and food necessarily assume some form of energy supply. The Inquiry was unable to obtain information as to how such supplies would be organised following an attack. In a nuclear attack oil would be especially vulnerable, even more than in a conventional attack.

Personal health

After a nuclear attack, those who had survived the effects of blast and thermal radiation and the early effects of nuclear radiation would next be exposed to lack of shelter, uncertain water supply, malnutrition and the risk of infection. There are several reasons why communicable diseases are likely to assume immediate importance. Many of the survivors would have been exposed to levels of radiation which are not sufficient to kill them outright, but which would have the effect of depressing their resistance to infection. There is experimental evidence that radiation may decrease the effectiveness of some mediative defence mechanisms, decrease the effectiveness of immunisation and cause a reduction in antibody response. People may be forced to cluster together around surviving facilities and this crowding might in itself promote the spread of infectious disease.

Diarrhoeal conditions

Recent investigations have shown that in a western country, such as the UK the common organisms which may cause diarrhoea and which are harboured by carriers are neither Salmonella typhi and Salmonella paratyphi, nor cholera, which can be highly life-threatening in the absence of chemotherapy. The common pathogens are a variety of other infectious agents for which often no anti-bacterial agents are appropriate. These infections carry a severe risk of dehydration. The effects of dehydration can be combated effectively by early and energetic oral rehydration with clean water containing sugar, i.e. glucose, dextrose or sucrose (20 g/litre), and common table salt, sodium chloride (3.5 g/litre). These additives to potable water are readily available in households and it is important that supplies of the two substances should be available. The Government booklets 'Protect and Survive'[32] and 'Domestic Nuclear Shelters'[17] list pure water and sugar for stocking shelters, but not salt. This omission should be rectified at once, perhaps with some advice on the composition of a salt and sugar fluid to prevent the onset of dehydration in diarrhoeas under shelter conditions.

Experience in treating diarrhoeas in the field in Third World countries has established that rehydration by oral 'salt and sugar water' is not only an effective lifesaving treatment but can be administered by parents, provided an effort to 'educate' them is undertaken. In the western world, with high technology medicine widely available, home rehydration is a concept little understood by most families. It is anticipated that intravenous rehydration would only be required in severe vomiting and diarrhoea.

It is of prime importance that the general public should attempt to ensure as high a standard of personal and food handling as is possible in a nuclear emergency and that the public should avoid faecal contamination of food, which is likely to be consumed cold in the absence of cooking facilities in shelter conditions.

Nevertheless, doctors would need to be vigilant—lest pathogens which require antibacterial drugs as well as rehydration become widespread. Such agents could spread from an unrecognised and untreated typhoid carrier, but this sort of hazard would be at the bottom of the list of the bacterial differential diagnoses unless an enemy indulged in bacterial warfare.

We consider that under field conditions, as in civilian practice, an untreated person with diarrhoea could cause widespread infection in large, closed communities. But most cases of diarrhoea in family shelters would be capable of effective shelter treatment by oral rehydration without intravenous and/or antibacterial drugs. It is unfortunate that similar simple measures applicable to the other grave medical conditions which may arise in the aftermath of a nuclear explosion would not be available to those in family shelters.

If an attack occurred in winter then many 'survivors' would be faced with the threat of hypothermia. It would be impossible to conduct immunisation campaigns against measles. Pertussis and diphtheria as well as poliomyelitis could spread in non-immunised infants. It is possible that diseases such as rheumatic fever which have fallen to a very low incidence in the developed world, would reappear.

Emerging from their shelters, survivors would face a major threat of bacterial infection — one moreover which could be expected to increase as the levels of radiation fell away. The 'classic' bacteria would be likely to cause epidemics of typhoid, paratyphoid, cholera and other enteric infectious diseases. Viral infections might also be common and, since insects are comparatively radiation-resistant, the proliferation of insects by which disease can be transmitted (insect vectors) might cause the reappearance in some countries of diseases such as typhus and malaria. Breakdown of rabies control is anticipated in those territories where the disease is present.

The survivors of a nuclear attack would probably spend between 14 and 21 days sheltering from the effects of radioactive fall-out. The Working Party believes that it is unlikely that outbreaks of diseases such as typhoid or cholera would occur during this period; there would be a higher probability of epidemics when survivors emerged from shelter and started to mix in larger groups.

Tuberculosis was a major cause of death in the 19th century and previous experience has shown an increased incidence of this disease in wartime. In World War II the death rate from tuberculosis rose 268 per cent in Berlin and 222 per cent in Warsaw. Thirty per cent, or just over 2000 survivors of the Dachau concentration camp, showed evidence of tuberculosis at the time of its liberation and in 40 per cent of these the disease was far advanced. In the event of nuclear war, the increase could be dramatic because of crowding and depressed levels of resistance due to radiation.

Psychiatric effects

The flood disaster in Bristol in 1968 brought an increase of 53 per cent in visits to doctors over the ensuing year. People who had suffered the greatest flood damage or who had required relocation showed the most significant increase in attendance. In this same year, too, hospital referrals and admissions were more than doubled for victims of the flood.

In addition to the immediate and relatively short-term psychological effects following a nuclear war it is likely that there would be some long-term effects. A delayed hazard of radiation is an increased incidence of cancer for which in many cases there could be no effective treatment. Survivors would also be burdened with the knowledge that succeeding generations might be harmed.

Long-term effects of radiation

Although the follow-up of certain exposed groups has left no doubt that radiation poses a carcinogenic risk, there are a variety of reasons why the exact magnitude of that risk has not yet been quantified. Often the exact dose of radiation received by exposed groups examined for the development of cancer has not been measured. The numbers of people developing cancer have been in many cases small and therefore confidence in any estimates has been limited. Other factors complicating the estimation of the cancer hazard from radiation include the long latent period for solid tumours and the difficulties of extrapolating from high- to low-dose exposure. It is generally agreed that there is no threshold for the carcinogenic effects of radiation.

There appears to be a difference between leukaemia and solid tumours with regard to the latent period between exposure to radiation and the development of clinical signs. The incidence of leukaemia reached a peak between six and seven years after the Japanese bombs and tended to decline thereafter. However, the incidence among exposed individuals between 1965 and 1971 was still higher than among the non-exposed population. Acute myeloid leukaemia was more common but there also appeared to be an increase in chronic myeloid leukaemia, particularly in patients who were exposed at Hiroshima. The great majority of cases of leukaemia occurred in those who had been exposed to 1 Gy or more. People under 30 years of age at the time of exposure tended to have a higher incidence of leukaemia occurring relatively soon after the event. However, in older victims, the increased incidence persisted longer, so that over the period 1950–1971 the incidence was similar over different age groups. The latency period for solid tumours following radiation exposure is considerably greater than that for leukaemia, averaging around 25 years.

There is evidence both from survivors of the bombings in Japan and from studies of Marshall islanders exposed in the 1954 Bravo test explosion that the incidence of thyroid cancer has increased. Of 86 islanders exposed to a radiation dose of between 1.35 and 11.5 Gy, thirty-one developed thyroid nodules between 1964 and 1979 and at least four developed thyroid cancer during this period. In addition, 13 of the 86 showed definite evidence of hypothyroidism with a further eight possible cases noted.

Other malignant conditions which have been found to increase in incidence following radiation exposure include breast cancer, lung cancer, malignant lymphoma, multiple myeloma, cancers of the gastro-intestinal tract and tumours of the salivary glands. According to figures given by the 1977 International Commission for Radiological Protection, total cancer mortality for exposure to 1 sievert (for gamma rays 1 sievert = 1 Gy) is one per cent. The actual incidence is likely to be considerably more than this since not all cancers are fatal. However, these figures are only rough estimates.

Genetic effects

Although a great deal is known about the genetics of radiation in animals there is still controversy about the effects in humans. The estimates of the doses required to double the natural mutation frequency in man vary from 0.16 Gy to 2.5 Gy. The effect of a 1 Gy exposure on the population could be to increase genetic abnormalities by 6% in the first generation and by 17% at equilibrium. Several studies have been performed on survivors of Hiroshima and Nagasaki showing chromosome aberrations in peripheral blood lymphocytes. In 1967 a study of 77 exposed survivors who were 30 or more years old at the time of atomic bomb exposure showed that when compared with 80 controls there was a significantly high frequency of radiation damage in the exposed. There is therefore no doubt that radiation caused long-term effects on chromosomes. However, the survivors as yet have shown no significant trend in the incidence of genetic effects except perhaps for an altered sex ratio.

CHAPTER 5

Home Defence

This chapter is about civil defence or home defence; the terms appear to us to be interchangeable. Civil defence in relation to a nuclear war would have to cover a range of organisational objectives dealing with the maintenance of a police function, the salvage of public utilities, transport and communications, in addition to questions affecting the common health of survivors. Both shelter building and evacuation policies have been expounded and criticised in the United States and we comment on designs for shelters that have been shown to the Working Party and report our discussions with a number of the experts who accepted invitations to meet members.

We have limited our inquiries to those aspects of civil defence that relate to the problems described in Chapters 3 and 4. Our comments are concerned directly with the reduction of casualty numbers and the provision of water, food, fuel, and shelter for the survivors.

An assessment of the value of civil defence was part of the task we were set by the ARM. Would a pattern of civil defence based on the experiences of World War II be effective, or would a nuclear attack be so quantitatively and qualitatively different as to invalidate previous assumptions and plans?

The concepts underlying civil defence arose out of the requirement to protect the population in World War II. World War II was remarkable because of the large-scale, repeated air attacks made against urban populations. Anxieties about the possibility of gas attacks required organisation both to distribute gas-masks of different types and to establish and maintain a monitoring and warning system.

Civil defence made a valuable and broadly successful contribution to limiting the damage caused by enemy attacks in World War II. Policies were evolved, for example on the transport of casualties to hospital, that increased the survival rate among casualties caused by high explosive bombs. The policy of splitting London and the Home Counties into four wedge-shaped sectors allowed personnel and materials to disperse to the countryside before an attack, returning to bring aid to damaged areas immediately afterwards.

The present plan

During any period of conventional war affecting the UK, the basic planning assumption is that the country would function as normally as possible for as long as possible. The Government envisages, however, that at a certain time in a period of tension preceding a nuclear attack, central Government would devolve its responsibilities to autonomous regional centres. Home Office circular ESC/1973 describes the machinery of government in war. Briefly, the system divides England into nine home defence regions, each containing one or more sub-regions. Commissioners for regions and sub-regions would be appointed to exercise the functions of government. Below sub-regional level, the processes of government would be carried out at county and district level. (In the capital, groups of London boroughs would equate to county level.) Each county and district has appointed a controller (designate) who would be empowered in war to exercise the full functions of government in his area. It is intended that a chain of government would be established from the region through to sub-region and county to district, supported by a network of communications.

The peacetime organisation of the National Health Service is not well suited to the likely needs of a decentralised government structure and we are told that it would be necessary to provide for a control structure through health service regions and districts to sectors and units for effective liaison with the appropriate region and sub-regions, and the county or district controller, at each level.

We were informed by Government that NATO policy generally is for the civil population to stay put in the event of hostilities and that this is the course which would be adopted in the UK. The Ministry of Defence agrees that in general terms 'it is fair to say that given the smallness of these islands and the strategic disposition of the various defence coponents, there are very few areas of the UK that do not have some defence basing'. There may be areas of the highlands of Scotland or Wales that would be immune from direct attack. The MoD spokesman went on to say that 'There are certainly large areas of the UK which, for strategic purposes, do have a very large number of defence bases'.

In relation to the question of evacuating civilians, the MoD spokesman said:

Unfortunately, one place is as unsafe as another in broad terms, and in all likelihood any attempts at mass evacuation would cause more problems than they would solve . . . . This is not a policy that is expected to be enforced. It is our advice to the public that they would do better in such a dreadful emergency to stay put and make shelter arrangements where they are.

The MoD spokesman emphasised that the role of the armed forces in the UK would be to act in support of the civil community as they do at present in major civilian disasters.

A plan has many levels. Parts of the civil defence plans used in World War II could still be relevant at a national level while other parts might be overtaken by the size of nuclear explosions or by a specific effect of a nuclear weapon such as the residual radioactivity following a ground-burst.

Part of the responsibility of decentralised Government at all levels would be to organise the suply of water and food to the survivors of a nuclear attack.

We are in no doubt that plans to encourage individuals to store adequate supplies of clean water and, similarly, the advice to paint a light coloured paint on house windows might indeed reduce the incidence of fires in houses on the fringes of an explosion by reducing the thermal radiation entering rooms. These elements of planning—the personal, individual precautions, that could be taken—have merit. This advice could prevent some of the short-term problems outlined in Chapter 3.

However, it appears to the Working Party that most of the Government's civil defence planning relates either to conventional warfare or to a small, isolated nuclear explosion. In the circumstances such as the 'average' attack postulated in Chapter 2 we doubt that the organisation and management implicit in the Government's plans would prove to be effective in the post-attack phase.

It appears to the Working Party that few people in the NHS understand what plans have been made for the Health Service in time of war (Chapter 6). A similar conclusion is difficult to avoid in terms of the problems identified by the Working Party in Chapter 4. The location of food dumps is not widely known and if there were to be a breakdown in the organisation set up by the Government then access to whatever limited food stores were available might be lost.

The delivery of the single daily meal of stew to survivors that is part of the Government's planning would require the collection of food, water, fuel, cooking and eating utensils into one place and organisation to prepare and distribute the meal. Experience of the relief of a number of concentration camps at the end of the World War II leads us to believe that people who are starving are not rational. Control of such a situation requires the presence of a strong or rational force. In addition to the opinion expressed by the MoD spokesman, the Home Office has said publicly that it is not intended that force will be used to control the actions of survivors.

Feeding children, people with diabetes and other special dietary requirements would present, we believe, insuperable problems. Such people would, in the words of the Home Office representative, 'have to fend for themselves'.

Many patients are now dependent on one or more public utilities for their survival outside hospital. Renal dialysis at home is a good example of skilled management applied to health care. A person using an artificial kidney machine requires a supply of about 40 gallons of pure water (at an adequate pressure) about two or three times each week. At present, water authorities notify patients in their area if there is to be a cessation of the supply or if maintenance work is to be carried out that might affect the water supply.

The plans that we know of for civil defence do not appear to take account of the dreadful psychological shock that would certainly affect the survivors of a major nuclear attack on the UK. We do not wish to underestimate any part of the damage, destruction and loss inflicted in the course of the World War II; however, there is no doubt that experience of conventional warfare is *irrelevant* to the scene that would confront whatever survivors remained after a major nuclear attack.

If the population is to stay put and exist largely on its own resources after a nuclear attack, what help may a family or individuals derive from a shelter? Beyond doubt, the effects of any nuclear weapon compared with those of a large conventional World War II bomb are so different that there is no point in attempting to judge shelter requirements or effectiveness by World War II standards. The impression we gained from the Home Office publications (*Protect and Survive*[32] and *Domestic Nuclear Shelters: Technical Guidance*)[17] is that both indoor and garden trench shelters are intended mainly to protect against fall-out in the post-attack phase. The protective factor of various shelter designs against radioactive fall-out is discussed in Chapter 3; however, the blast protection offered by shelters which are easily constructed is minimal.

A simple shelter (Type 1a) for short term (say 10-14 days') use can be built using materials already at hand about the home. It is based upon a trench in the garden 18 inches deep and 15 feet in length. The trenching soil is used to raise 24 inch walls to support doors as roofing and the whole is protected by a covering of earth domed up at least

18 inches high. These simply constructed, cramped quarters are expected to remain intact at a distance of seven or more miles beyond a one-megaton explosion, affording blast and fall-out protection.

Another improvised outdoor shelter (Type 1b) is tent-shaped and uses alloy or steel tubular scaffold poles to support a plywood roof with earth cover. It is based on a trench 8 feet by 8 feet and 18 inches deep and is expected to remain intact beyond three miles of ground zero.

The simple types 1a and 1b might give some protection against blast. They should not be expected to do more than offer some protection against radiation utilizing on-site materials. More substantial shelters could give better blast and fall-out protection, but in the Government and commercial designs shown to the Working Party, ventilation is maintained by mechanical pump systems which rely on the ability of the inmates to turn a handle either continuously or at required intervals. None of the pump ventilation systems seem to be able to eliminate combustion products emitted by fires on the surface outside the shelter. The filters in the pumps might trap smoke particles, although this is doubtful, but they would not be effective in removing gaseous contaminants which could threaten the lives of the inmates. The air intake vent on at least one model of buried shelter could be vulnerable to blast and debris.

Civil defence has been scrutinised intensely in the United States. We were fortunate that Professor Bernard Lown and Dr David Greer were able to come to Britain to discuss questions about civil defence with the Inquiry.

Professor Lown: 'The major question in the US is about a plan of evacuation. The evaluation has largely abandoned shelters as a motive for civil defence; that was thought through and discredited'.

BMA: 'We may be talking about shelters in different ways. What does a shelter mean to you?'

Professor Lown: 'A shelter varies from individual shelters that individuals may build in their cellars to shelters in tunnels or subways for public accommodation. This underlies the concept of Federal Emergency Management Agency (FEMA) because it is pointed out that shelters in big cities are designed in the absence of a fire storm. There is not going to be any shelter because that has been abandoned, with the exception of the heavy blast centres for works in industries that cannot be evacuated . . . . A shelter policy is so costly the US Government is not going to be involved in that.'

BMA: 'The current policy in this country is that people should stay put because apart from anything else if you evacuate people you destroy the country's industrial activity very effectively. That is as effective as dropping bombs. Where are people evacuated to? You have wide open areas, but not all of them are hospitable.'

Professor Lown: 'Evacuation is very arbitrary. Boston moves partially to Cape Cod and Greenfield, Massachusetts, but there are residents in Greenfield who say, we will not have it. Not only that, but how do you move people? On Friday you are paralysed with people going out for the weekend . . . . Who says there is going to be time? Let us assume there will be time, and we move 80 per cent of the population. In the United States it would cost $6 billion per day in lost productivity. This is the calculated cost. If anyone wants to put a country out of business you do not have to drop bombs—evacuation would have the same effect. That means that moving out people compels pre-emption . . . .

'We have discussed several factors where civil defence does not become a way of saving people, it becomes a war measure of hastening the Doomsday which everyone says they are trying to avoid . . . .

'Look what happened at Three Mile Island. That is an important lesson to look at carefully. There was a period of 60 minutes where meltdown seemed likely. The cost of evacuating people becomes enormous, and the Government of Pennsylvania evacuated only pregnant women . . . . Supposing it is winter time, who in his right mind is going to go out in the savage wild? Supposing it is summer, who is going to go out in the desert without a water supply?'

Planning for emergencies

Annex 5 sets out overall plans for dealing with emergencies at nuclear reactor plants in the UK. We note that an emergency at a plant or in the course of transporting nuclear material occurs at a known geographical location or along a defined route. Nuclear reactors cannot explode and although a catastrophic meltdown might release large quantities of radioactive material, there would be no blast or heat damage of the sort associated with a nuclear explosion. Yet elaborate planning and organisation have been carried out so that the authorities would be in a position to minimise the effects of a reactor incident.

Provision is made for evacuation of people threatened by fall-out from a catastrophic meltdown. Road transport would not be affected as there would be no blast damage to roads or buildings and fuel and electricity supplies would remain largely uninterrupted. Communications networks would be intact. All of these facilities are essential if the present plans for an emergency at a nuclear power plant are to be effective. We believe that such plans for a major civilian disaster have every chance of success and should be strongly supported by the medical profession. The profession has a duty to involve itself in planning for emergencies of this nature.

Compare the uninterrupted peacetime conditions that we have described with the devastation outlined in Chapters 2 and 3. It becomes clear that breakdown to be expected in transport and communications systems alone would prevent any possibility of effective planning on a national or regional scale. Uncertainty about the targets for a nuclear attack coupled with the massive destruction caused even by small 'tactical' weapons means that any attempt to lay plans for medical services, food supplies for all possible nuclear emergencies becomes a myth.

The shelters advocated by the Government and commercial suppliers may improve the chance of survival for some people in the short term but the overwhelming problems of infection, bacterial contamination of water and the scarcity of food and fuel would still remain to be faced when the survivors emerged.

A shelter policy has been abandoned in the United States and the current evacuation policy is under attack for being impractical. The intermixing of potential targets and population centres in the UK makes an evacuation policy even less viable here. The current advice by Government to stay where you live and work acknowledges this fact. There is no place on the UK mainland that could be guaranteed to be free from the effects of a nuclear attack.

CHAPTER 6

The Health Service

*The Government and health authorities have published plans for the
National Health Service in time of war. These plans are examined
alongside predictions for differing patterns of nuclear attack and
projections for the resulting numbers of casualties. Serious deficiencies,
which may be inevitable due to the uncertainties inherent in any
nuclear attack, are highlighted.*

Government assumptions in planning

Government planning for war is based on a period of escalating international tension during which there might be conventional bombing of
selected military targets in the UK. During this period plans would be
implemented in preparation for a partial or all-out nuclear attack.
Current planning is based largely on the problems resulting from the
nuclear attack phase. Assessments of the length of the period of international tension have been progressively reduced from three weeks to
four days. We have been told that the general aim of current
Government planning is to avoid disrupting the economic and
industrial life of the country for as long as possible. The Government
says that the aim of the Health Service would be to provide such
medical and nursing care as is practicable for casualties of war and for
the sick, as well as providing a basic structure for the future reconstruction of health and other social services.

The Department of Health and Social Security circular HDC(77)1:
The Preparation and Organisation of the Health Service for War
(issued in 1977 and reproduced in Annex 6) directs health authorities
to plan to meet the consequences of a nuclear attack on any part
of the country, including direct attack, radioactive fall-out hazards,
problems resulting from the movement of the population and the
interruption of supplies. The essence of these plans is devolution from
central Government to administration in nine specified home defence
regions.

112

DHSS responsibilities and medical plans for civil defence

The DHSS is responsible for all aspects of the health services, for local authority personal social services and for social security. In the context of civil defence DHSS personal social services would be concerned with such matters as assistance to those rendered destitute or homeless and to refugees, while social security would continue in its normal form, or in a modified form for as long as possible—until, for example, the monetary system broke down. DHSS representatives have said in discussion with the Working Party that the health services would seek to play a vital role in all stages of the emergency—transition to war, the period of hostilities, and the aftermath of war.

The Government assumption is that during any period of conventional hostilities affecting the UK, the country would function as normally as possible and that no large-scale reorganisation of the NHS would occur. However, during the period of tension prior to the declaration of war, health authorities would aim to reduce hospital populations as far as possible to provide space for casualties of conventional fighting in Europe and the UK. Beds would become available following the discharge of patients as set out in the DHSS circular.

The DHSS says that the ability of the NHS to cope with the effects of a 'conventional' bombardment would depend upon the nature, severity and frequency of the attacks. A limited number of casualties within a given area might not overstretch the resources of the local hospital, whereas a larger incident would invoke the health authority's major disaster plan, bringing in other hospitals and more on-site resources. In areas where a larger number of incidents is anticipated it might be necessary to expand the major disaster plan, especially with regard to transport of patients and supply of additional resources.

NHS wartime role

The point at which the NHS would assume its wartime role depends on decisions made by central Government about the devolution of its function to a regional organisation. Briefly, the arrangement is that England would be divided into nine home defence regions, each containing one or more sub-regions (which are not necessarily co-terminous with existing parts of the NHS structure). Commissioners would be appointed for regions and sub-regions to exercise the functions of government. Below sub-region, the process of government would be carried out at county and district level. (In London, groups of London boroughs would constitute county levels.) Each county and district would have a controller empowered in war to exercise the full functions of government in his area. A chain of government could thus be established from the region through to sub-region, county and district, supported by a network of communications.

An independent communications system is in existence to connect emergency sub-regional headquarters, with links to the counties and districts. This consists of private underground telephone cables (also capable of carrying teleprinter traffic) and a radio communications system.

The DHSS circular states:

The peacetime administrative structure of the Health Service is unsuited to the needs of war, when a clear system of control would be needed for the rapid acquisition and redeployment of surviving resources. A control structure would be required which could be activated before an attack and which would relate to the various levels of wartime regional government.

Health authorities have been advised by the DHSS each to appoint a health director (designate) who would assume wartime responsibilities for all the authority's functions.

The scope for further dispersing the ambulance service is probably limited, but authorities have been asked to plan to disperse vehicles so that an emergency radio network might be established using whatever equipment survives. The dispersal of staff from central urban areas has been considered and the current advice is that, as soon as patients have been sent home, all staff not required to operate an emergency service should be sent home or dispersed widely within the region.

In evidence given to the Working Party by the DHSS it is stated that the probable effect of a nuclear attack on the organisation described above is difficult to assess. If all the elements of planning have been achieved then it would be reasonable to expect that in any area where there were survivors there would be some kind of health care, albeit basic and limited in capacity. The DHSS notes that in some places there could be no recognisable health care provision remaining after a major attack, but considers that it would be inhumane not to make plans in advance to care for survivors wherever possible.

The DHSS states that:

When movement became possible, emphasis would have to be placed on self-help, with minor injuries being treated by relatives or friends, to avoid over-burdening the health services with cases of superficial injury. More serious casualties would be treated at First Aid Posts (FAPs), established by the

Voluntary Aid Societies. Casualties requiring further treatment would be sent to nearby Casualty Collecting Centres (CCCs) run by general medical practitioners with the assistance of the Domiciliary Teams and volunteers. CCCs would treat and sort casualties for priority admission to hospital, return to the community or temporary retention. The resources available to the health services however would dictate that the majority of casualties would have to be cared for by relatives, friends or volunteers, in their own homes or local authority rest centres, with assistance from general practitioners and members of the Domiciliary Teams based on the CCCs.

The DHSS believes that during a period of crisis individuals with a knowledge of first aid would volunteer their services. They would be directed to a voluntary aid society which would allocate them to a first aid post close to their homes. A national appeal would be made for all those with medical or nursing qualifications (but not currently practising) to report to their nearest casualty collecting centre as soon as possible.

The DHSS has told the Working Party that it will be necessary, in the near future, to revise and reissue Circular HDC(77)1, originally issued in 1977, to take account of the 1980 review of home defence and, perhaps more crucially as far as the Health Service is concerned, the restructured NHS.

As an example of how the Department's strategy has been translated into concrete terms, the preparatory requirements established by the East Anglian Regional Health Authority for an emergency transfusion service are as follows:

1 Increase present stocks of plastic packs for blood collection from four to at least six months. Also explore the possibility of re-establishing stocks of reusable equipment.
2 Agree on siting of district transfusion services and nominate a hospital transfusion officer and staff. Assess hospital equipment and accommodation for collection, testing and storage.
3 Accommodation for Blood Transfusion Services staff and equipment which might be dispersed pre-strike.
4 Peacetime recruitment and training of voluntary nursing staff.
5 Peacetime training of some hospital staff in blood transfusion techniques.
6 Peacetime training of selected SRNs for blood collection.
7 Powers to commandeer at short notice from pre-strike phase onwards:
   (a) suitable premises for blood donors (schools, church halls, etc)
   (b) means of publicity — radio, television, loudspeakers
   (c) additional vehicles during pre-strike fighting phase and post-strike.

8 Guidance on powers of command and direction of staff during emergency and war conditions.
9 Advice on the fitness for blood donation of volunteers exposed to radiation.

Role of voluntary organisations

County authorities are responsible for recruiting, training and organising volunteers for home defence. The DHSS anticipates that the voluntary aid societies (St John's Ambulance Brigade, St Andrew's Ambulance Association and British Red Cross Society) will play a major role in staffing First Aid Posts.

Discussions on a home defence role have led to some change of emphasis in training objectives. The Working Party was told that it is obviously important, against the background of a nuclear attack, to increase the emphasis on collective training. This involves integrating first aid and nursing personnel into composite rescue teams capable of adapting themselves rapidly to a disaster, dealing with mass casualties and supervising the work of other volunteers, many of whom will have minimal training.

Women's Royal Voluntary Service (WRVS)

This organisation has local volunteer groups in existence in peacetime and in many places they take on the responsibility for providing such services as meals-on-wheels. It is expected that they will play a major part in emergency feeding in the post-attack. The WRVS already has 570 depots of secondhand clothing.

The DHSS stressed in oral evidence to us that medical services for war are currently intended initially to provide for a period of conventional warfare. We can see the wisdom of making plans of this nature, and it is possible that, if such a system were fully operational, it might give a community peripheral to the target area a better chance of surviving some of the effects of a nuclear attack.

On the other hand, the wording of the present circular, which clearly shows conventional warfare to be merely a prelude to a nuclear attack, deals with the situation following a nuclear attack.

We remain strongly of the view that the medical profession has a responsibility to involve itself in contingency planning to meet a wide variety of major disasters. Elements of this experience might then benefit some survivors in some areas following a nuclear attack.

The principal deficiency of present planning is that the range of offensive options available to an enemy is so wide that it is impracticable to envisage arrangements to cover them all. The current DHSS circular refers to contingency planning for a period of conventional warfare but almost immediately launches into the need for plans to cover nuclear exchange.

Many witnesses to the Working Party expressed the view that, apart from a single demonstration attack—recognised as such by both sides—an exchange of nuclear weapons would quickly lead to a massive nuclear attack on the UK. While there would undoubtedly be survivors (and the survival rate could be improved by contingency planning), the sheer scale of the nuclear threat makes it difficult to comprehend the outcome. Civilised life as we know it, and the human values and ethical standards upon which the practice of medicine is based would cease to exist in vast areas of these islands. It would be impossible to run even a basic medical care service without minimal standards of law and order. Survivors would be preoccupied exclusively with the search for food and shelter. They would be unlikely to devote attention to the care of the sick and dying.

It must be assumed that NHS personnel will have suffered the same fate as the rest of the population. Their preoccupations are likely to be the paramount ones of personal and family survival. We do not doubt that doctors would wish to give help even in the midst of such devastation, nor do we doubt that they would be looked upon by survivors as natural leaders; but their impact on the situation would be minimal.

The creation of emergency organisations assumes that the identified personnel will be available but they too are likely to have suffered in the general destruction. The present rigid structures which are being prepared in response to the DHSS circular will be ineffective in a situation of mass devastation following a major nuclear attack. There is no guarantee that key personnel would be able to fulfil the tasks allotted to them. The probability is that many would not.

We are not convinced that the overwhelming priority of doctors and nurses in such a situation should be to rebuild the previously existing medical services. There will be better prospects for survival of the community if priority is given to the provision of food and shelter and to basic public health measures such as the digging of latrines and the identification of clean water sources. It is these priorities which should be urged on the relevant professions now if planning for this scale of devastation is to be undertaken. When some rudimentary medical services are re-established, doctors will find themselves forced by necessity to carry out some procedures which they have not undertaken for many years, if ever.

There remains a possible scenario for which planning might be effective. This is the 'demonstration attack' using a single nuclear weapon. How realistic such a scenario might be we have no means of assessing, but on the evidence we have received this would carry the risk of escalation. The situation would be like that of Hiroshima, where a particular locality was subjected to nuclear bombardment. The affected area could expect substantial and powerful support within a relatively short time after the attack. The point of disaster planning in this context is not one of self-help within the devastated area, but the mobilisation of personnel and resources to bring in medical services, food, water and shelter from outside. A key difference following the detonation of a single nuclear weapon is that national services would be largely intact.

Our conclusions about the number of casualties resulting from the explosion of a single nuclear weapon over a UK population centre have been reported and should be set against the possibility of taking aid into an area affected by a nuclear explosion, or of removing casualties from it. The present arrangements, particularly for health service planning, are far too rigid, identifying specific individuals and allocating specific roles to groups of personnel for situations which may prove in the event to be radically different from those envisaged.

Our attention has been drawn to other forms of training which seem to have more to offer in such situations. In our view, the natural leaders who emerge will be those with problem-solving skills. Since the specific problems cannot be foreseen beforehand the ability to identify a problem and to suggest solutions from the resources immediately to hand are likely to be more valuable than the bureaucratic skills envisaged in following orders through a chain of command which may no longer exist.

Problem-solving is of course the essence of the medical art applied to patients. The approach taken in medical training does, however, encourage the student to consider every possibility and to eliminate each one in turn. This is somewhat different from the skill of identifying the easiest and most probable solution and then moving on to others as each solution proves inadequate. It is these skills in problem-solving which should feature large in any preparation of the profession to deal with disasters. We should like to see training designed to encourage doctors to review their roles in such situations and to assess priorities and objectives.

Comments on current DHSS plans

It seems to us that the present planning arrangements for the health services in time of nuclear war are seriously deficient in important respects.

The current DHSS circular deals with planning both for conventional and for nuclear warfare, but these two threads are tangled. The DHSS has indicated that they intend to revise HDC(77)1 and this revision may necessitate modifications of our comments. In the meantime our comments are:

1 There is apparent confusion over suggested medical requirements in conventional and nuclear warfare.
2 The needs of each are opposed in certain important respects. Conventional warfare demands the concentration of facilities and expertise, whereas both should be dispersed as widely as possible before a nuclear attack.
3 The scale of devastation in nuclear war could make current suggested patterns of organisation inappropriate.
4 The planning requirements for conventional and for nuclear warfare diverge in important respects because of the magnitude of areas of damage and casualties. The Inquiry feels that the two planning requirements should be kept separate. In conventional warfare experience indicates that medical facilities broadly follow peacetime patterns. In nuclear warfare these facilities would be largely destroyed.

CHAPTER 7

Summary and conclusions

This chapter of the report gives a dispassionate summary of the medical consequences that would follow the explosion of nuclear weapons over the United Kingdom.

We repeat that we have formed our judgements about the effects of nuclear war on the basis of the information and evidence presented to us. Each reader will make up his own mind on matters connected with the nuclear weapons debate.

Nuclear war affecting the United Kingdom

The UK contains a large number of targets likely to be attacked in war and has densely populated conurbations. Potential targets and population centres are intermixed across the UK so that it is not possible to discern areas, apart from remote tracts in Scotland, and perhaps in North Wales, that do not place potential targets adjacent to communities of people.

The population density of the UK is 593 people per square mile. England has a higher density of 920 people per square mile. The population density coupled with the number and distribution of potential targets is unique to the UK. No other country has so many people and so many potential targets concentrated into so small a land mass.

In the 1960s aggregation of world nuclear weapons of an explosive power of 400 megatons was thought to ensure deterrence by Mutually Assured Destruction of both the USA and the USSR essential targets. Estimates of the total explosive power of world nuclear arsenals in 1980 varied between 25 and 50 times that quantity (10,000-20,000 megatons). Any realistic assessment of the medical effects of nuclear war must take into account changes in technology and military strategy. The effects of an attack in 1950 would have been very different from the effects of an attack now or in the future.

120

None of the organisations or individuals who sent papers to the Working Party, or who gave oral presentations, were able to predict with certainty where an attack on the UK with nuclear weapons would occur or what form such an attack would take. The unreliability of basic assumptions has been a constantly recurring problem in all areas of our investigation. Uncertainty in areas of our report is inevitable; nobody has direct experience of a nuclear attack of the magnitude envisaged in the future. However, both Government and independent authorities have suggested that an attack could well be of the order of 200 megatons or greater. Furthermore, with one exception, all the experts who contributed to the Working Party said that a nuclear war could not be contained, but would escalate to an unlimited, total exchange of nuclear weapons.

There are discrepancies between the projections for blast, heat and radiation produced by the Home Office and Scientists Against Nuclear Arms (SANA). The latter rely on methods and figures derived for the most part from the United States Department of Defense and the Office of Technology Assessment. We have examined the methods for calculating the projections used by SANA and the Working Party believes, on the evidence it has received, that the projections from SANA give a more realistic estimate of the blast, heat and radiation effects of nuclear weapons. We understand that the Home Office is currently revising its calculations.

Civil defence — evacuation

Evacuation policies have their problems. Sufficient warning is needed in order to evacuate successfully. The economic cost to the country is tremendous and for these reasons governments would be very unwilling to put evacuation plans into practice. If, however, an attempt was made to evacuate the general population, this would be seen by an enemy as part of preparations for war and might invite a pre-emptive strike.

Given the uncertainty about the pattern of an attack, that is the number and size of weapons, where they would be detonated, and the period of time over which the explosions would occur, evacuation is impossible in the UK. The Government's advice to stay where you are, at home, at work or at school, effectively acknowledges this fact. There is no point upon the surface of the UK mainland that could be guaranteed immune from the effects of nuclear attacks.

Civil defence — shelters

The makeshift home shelters advocated by the Home Office would offer the occupants only slight protection against the blast emitted by an exploding nuclear weapon. Burns and injuries caused by flying glass from shattered windows could be reduced but there would be little protection against radioactive fall-out. Repeated explosions would diminish the protection against fall-out.

Advice to site the shelter at the central core of a house or building carries the risk that a substantial proportion of domestic shelters are likely to be buried when the surrounding dwelling collapses. No heavy rescue services would be available to excavate trapped survivors. If the shelter was situated near an outside wall, the occupants would be more at risk from the fall-out.

In a large-scale nuclear attack many areas of the country would be subjected to levels of blast damage sufficient to destroy these improvised shelters. The greater part of the country would experience blast pressures sufficient to break windows or remove doors or roof tiles from houses, which would in turn limit the protection provided against fall-out. This factor is not allowed for in the current Home Office calculations.

Some of the commercially available prefabricated domestic nuclear shelters could offer a degree of protection against blast and heat and all would protect against fall-out. None of the designs reported to the Working Party appears to have satisfactory mechanisms to eliminate dangerous combustion products of the air being drawn into the shelter. A large-scale programme of public shelter building would be very costly. It could be effective in reducing short-term casualties. Any survivors would face overwhelming problems in the world into which they emerged.

Long-term effects of a nuclear attack

Water would be the first requirement of survivors of a nuclear attack. Food, shelter, fossil fuels and electrical power would follow in order of priority. The present water tanker capacity in the UK is wholly inadequate to supply survivors with water for even basic needs. Government plans for the supply and distribution of emergency supplies of food do not aim to provide a balanced diet. This would have serious consequences for people requiring special diets, diabetic patients, for example. There may not be a sufficient quantity of food in store to tide survivors over until alternative sources could be found.

Survivors would have to change their dietary patterns to include a much greater amount of diverse cereals and vegetables. Palatability of food that might be available would be a major problem. Water and fuel are necessary to render many cereals edible.

There is a probability that the atmosphere would be highly perturbed by a nuclear war. The large quantities of highly sunlight-absorbing, dark particulate matter which would be produced and spread in the troposphere by the many fires would strongly restrict the penetration of sunlight to the earth's surface and would change the physical properties of the earth's atmosphere. It is likely that agricultural production in the Northern Hemisphere would be severely disrupted, so that food production for the survivors of the initial effects of the war would be very difficult.

Survival becomes even more difficult if stratospheric ozone depletions also take place. It is difficult to see how much more than a small fraction of the initial survivors of a nuclear war in the middle and high latitude regions of the Northern Hemisphere could escape famine and disease during the following years.

Other problems with implications for public health would be extensive radioactive contamination of the environment, failure of water and sewerage systems and lack of basic drugs and medical supplies.

It is inaccurate and misleading to suggest that after a nuclear attack on the United Kingdom there would be a return to a rural civilisation of two centuries ago. The Working Party believes that there would be an increase in infant mortality, communicable diseases due to infections, and deficiency diseases caused by inadequate nutrition. The UK no longer possesses the skills or primitive technologies which allowed our predecessors an existence with some measure of comfort. The skills of the 20th century do not permit a return to that style of life after a nuclear attack.

Effects on medical services

We cannot forecast what sizes of weapons might be exploded over the UK. Most current strategic and intermediate range or theatre weapons have explosive yields of between 100 kilotons and 5 megatons. The bomb dropped at Hiroshima was between 12-20 kilotons in size.

The extent of damage caused by a nuclear weapon does not increase in direct proportion to the explosive yield. Thus, to double the distance at which a given level of damage is caused requires an eight-fold increase in explosive power. It follows that if a given total weight of attack is divided into a larger number of smaller weapons, greater damage will be caused. The argument sometimes advanced that more accurate lower yield weapons will result in fewer casualties is a false one, so long as the total explosive power used in an attack remains similar.

The explosion of a single nuclear bomb of the size used at Hiroshima over a major city in the UK is likely to produce so many cases of trauma and burns requiring hospital treatment that the remaining medical services in the UK would be completely overwhelmed. An attack with, for example, 200 megatons represents an explosive power some 15,000 times greater than the Hiroshima bomb; or the equivalent of forty (40) times all the conventional explosive used in the whole of the Second World War.

The NHS could not deal with the casualties that might be expected following the detonation of a single one megaton weapon over the UK. It follows that multiple nuclear explosions over several, possibly many, cities would force a breakdown in medical services across the country as a whole.

There is no possibility of increasing the production of certain drugs in a short period of tension before a war, and if we wish to have large quantities of blood products available for transfusion purposes or the bulk of the present generation of medical practitioners in the country trained for certain eventualities, then all of these things would have to be done now and the country must exist on a more or less permanent emergency footing.

We believe that such a weight of nuclear attack would cause the medical services in the country to collapse. The provision of individual medical or nursing attention for victims of a nuclear attack would become remote. At some point it would disappear completely and only the most primitive first aid services might be available from a fellow survivor.

Board of Science and Education
terms of reference

1.   To advise and, when so empowered, to act for the Council in all matters, not specifically referred to a committee of the Association, which concern the work of the Association for the promotion of the medical and allied sciences. In particular to advise and act in matters concerning: the Nuffield Library of the Association, the British Life Assurance Trust, the Film Library, Association Grants, Scholarships, Research Awards and Prizes.

2.   With the consent of Council, to initiate studies and to report with recommendations in matters of medical concern to the community or to the medical profession.

3.   To make a report to the Council annually, and at such other times as may be expedient on the matters for which it is responsible.

Organisations and individuals who submitted evidence

* Gave oral evidence

Dr Sheila Adam

Mr E. E. Alley

Arms Control and Disarmament Unit, the Foreign and Commonwealth Office*

Association of British Pharmaceutical Industries, Mr A. J. Badby, Mr A. Murray*

ASTMS

Mr S. Bailey

Dr J. H. Baumer

Professor I. Bellany

The Bishop of Salisbury*

Dr K. Boddy

Dr Mary E. Brennan

British Institute of Radiology, Technical Working Party, Professor J. Boag*

Dr S. Britten

Surg. Lt Cdr J. Bunyan

Centre for Configurational Studies, the Open University, Mr P. Steadman*

Dr J. E. Coggle

CONTACT

Dr B. G. Cowie

Dr J. M. Cundy

Department of Health and Social Security*

Ms T. A. Devereux

Dr S. Dowling

Dr P. Draper

Dr M. Eastwood

Mr P. Ekins

Dr F. Ellis

Dr I. W. Fingland

Dr S. Geisner

Major General R. J. Gray

Dr Jane Grubb

Dr A. Haines

Brigadier M. Harbottle

Dr M. Hartog

Harvard School of Public Health USA, Professor B. Lown*

The Home Office*

The Hope Medical Clinic

Mrs E. A. Horwell

Dr J. Hutchinson

Professor N. F. Kember

Dr Kirk

Mr E. Lambert

Dr J. Law

Dr R. H. Lawson

Dr K. Little

London School of Hygiene and Tropical Medicine

Dr H. A. R. Loxdale

Dr J. Marrow

Dr Sue McAlliou

Dr C. Mawdsley

Mr R. Meads

Medical Campaign Against Nuclear Weapons, Professor J. H. Humphrey, Dr B. Beaumont*

Dr H. Middleton

N. A. Minaur

The Ministry of Agriculture, Fisheries and Food

Ministry of Defence*

The National Radiologists Protection Board

Professor M. Pentz

Plessey Controls Ltd, Mr D. Higginbottom*

Dr A. Poteliakhoff

Reading University, Mr J. A. Burns, Mr L. Jollans, Mr E. C. Apling, Mr R. S. Taylor*

Regional Medical Officer, N. E. Thames Regional Health Authority

Dr P. Roberts

Dr J. R. Robinson

Dr M. Sharp

Mr A. B. Stinchcombe

Stockholm International Peace Research Institute, Dr F. Barnaby*

Dr A. Qasrawi

The UK Atomic Energy Authority

Dr P. R. Webber

Professor B. G. F. Weitz*

Dr H. Zealley

ANNEX 3

Articles from the
British Medical Journal

From: The *British Medical Journal*
1 February 1975, Vol 1, pp.256-259

Occasional survey

The Summerland disaster

R. J. Hart, J. O. Lee, D. J. Boyles, N. R. Batey

The reception, admission, and subsequent management of casualties from the Summerland fire are described. A senior member of the staff assessed priorities and directed casualties to different prearranged teams, and a nurse was allocated to each patient to aid continuity of treatment and documentation.

Though regular revision and discussion of major accident procedures with all members of the hospital staff and co-ordination with other rescue workers is helpful expensive reheasals are of limited value in a civilian incident.

Introduction

Some confusion is apt to occur in a non-specialized hospital when even a few patients with moderately serious burns are admitted as an emergency. The special care they need can impose considerable strain on the staff and the available facilities.

Noble's Hospital in Douglas is a general hospital which serves the 56,000 residents of the Isle of Man as well as the 500,000 yearly visitors. Of the 200 beds seven are in an intensive care unit formed six years ago. There is no separate burns unit as the number of seriously burnt patients treated is normally small. During the period August 1972 to

August 1973 155 patients with recent burns or scalds were treated in the casualty department and 12 were admitted. None needed resuscitation with intravenous fluids, and only two needed skin grafts.

On the evening of 2 August 1973 about 3000 people, mostly holiday-makers, were enjoying the facilities of the Summerland leisure complex. A fire, started in an adjacent kiosk, spread within minutes to engulf the whole building. During the rush towards the exits many were injured by being crushed or trampled upon, and others tried to jump to safety. Some were burnt as they tried to leave the building, and others inhaled smoke when returning to find lost relatives. Within minutes of the alarm being given casualties started to arrive at the hospital, brought by taxis and private cars as well as by ambulance. In response to radio appeals blood donors also arrived and the roads to the hospital were severely congested.

Reception of casualties

The initial problems were to mobilize the necessary staff and equipment and sort out the patients as they arrived at the casualty department. The telephone operator called both resident and non-resident staff in accordance with the emergency regulations, which fortunately had recently been revised. Indeed there was shortly more help than could be used as all the medical and nursing staff and many volunteers offered their services. Blood donors were assembled in a nearby hall and 44 pints of blood collected. Most of the patients and their relatives arrived within 20 minutes of the alarm being given and nearly all within an hour. The large number of people in the casualty department caused some confusion and made it difficult for the hospital staff to keep in contact and work effectively together.

Fatal injuries

Forty-eight people were dead on arrival at the hospital. The main causes of death were suffocation, carbon monoxide poisoning, burns, and multiple injuries from falling. A high proportion of the tracheae and bronchi contained soot. The 48 bodies were taken to the hospital mortuary and then to a nearby church hall where more space was available. They were labelled by letter, and necropsies were performed over the next three days. The process of identification continued over the following week, during which time the bodies were preserved without refrigeration in a polythene tube tied at both ends. The tube contained 200 ml of 4% formaldehyde and a similar quantity of formaldehyde injected intraperitoneally. Only 12 of the bodies were visually identifiable.

Positive identification was obtained in all cases but presented considerable problems. Property, such as jewellery and necklaces, was sometimes helpful. The final identification was by a combination of sex, approximate age, teeth (dentures or dental charts), and operations such as hysterectomy or caesarean section.

Non-fatal injuries

As they arrived at the hospital soon after the incident even the extensively burnt patients were not severely shocked. Intravenous infusions were set up in the casualty department and intravenous morphine or pethidine given where indicated. A nurse was allocated to each patient to help with documentation and continuity of treatment. Altogether 104 beds were made available, including five in the intensive care unit, by moving patients to day rooms. These patients were later discharged or accommodated elsewhere in the hospital.

Seventy patients with minor burns, fractures, lacerations and emotional stress were treated and followed up as outpatients. A total of 32 patients were admitted to hospital. Fourteen had a variety of injuries to the chest, abdomen, or limbs, including three with pelvic fractures. None of these injuries were serious. Most were admitted primarily for their burns.

ASPHYXIA

Three patients were admitted to the intensive therapy unit with asphyxia.

Case 1—A 51-year-old man had a long history of bronchitis and smoked 60 cigarettes daily. He was admitted direct from the fire semi-comatose and very restless. He was deeply cyanosed, severely dyspnoeic, and wheezy. A chest X-ray examination showed bilateral pulmonary oedema. His PCO_2 was 5.9 kPa (45 mm Hg).

Case 2—A man aged 18 had lost consciousness during the fire. He was trapped in a room near the top of the building for four hours after the start of the fire. His friend in the same room died but he had sat under a dripping tap with his jacket over his head. He was treated for apparent cardiac arrest on arrival at the casualty department and his circulation soon improved. He was deeply cyanosed with dyspnoea, pulmonary oedema, and bronchospasm. Chest X-ray examination showed bilateral pulmonary oedema. His PCO_2 was 5.5 kPa (41 mm Hg).

Case 3—A 56-year-old woman who had a history of chest trouble after influenza in 1971 had returned to her hotel after the fire, but the next day she became progressively wheezy and was admitted to hospital 18 hours later. A chest X-ray examination showed nothing abnormal and her PCO_2 was 5.9 kPa (45 m Hg).

Management

Hydrocortisone 100 mg intravenously was given every four to six hours. We felt that the need to relieve bronchospasm was greater than the need for any anti-inflammatory action of the steroid. Initially ampicillin was used as a broad-spectrum antibiotic but sputum was cultured daily for each patient and the drug changed when indicated. One patient (case 1) became infected with pseudomonas, and was treated with carbenicillin intravenously and by inhalation using an ultrasonic nebulizer.

Oxygen was given by facemask in an attempt to reduce the arterial desaturation. Sedation was necessary to relieve the initial restlessness in two of the patients. Diazepam 5 mg intravenously was given for its lack of respiratory depressant effect.

Blood gases were estimated often during the early stages. The PCO_2 in case 1 rose from 5.9 to 10.7 kPa (45 to 80 mm Hg) on the day after the fire. The patient was intubated and ventilated by intermittent positive pressure ventilation (IPPR). A tracheostomy was performed on the second day and IPPR continued for four days.

Vigorous chest physiotherapy was begun as soon as the patient became sufficiently co-operative. During their four sessions daily the three patients expectorated large quantities of black carbonaceous sputum for several days.

Progress was satisfactory in all three patients. One patient (case 3) was discharged after 14 days, one (case 1) after 17 days; and the last (case 2) after 19 days. Their subsequent respiratory progress continued to be satisfactory but at least one patient was troubled with recurrent nightmares of the disaster.

Table I— *Degree of Burns in 24 Patients admitted with Surface Burns*

Body surface burnt (%):	<10	10-20	-30	40-50	55	65
No. of patients	11	5	4	2	1	1
Outcome	Recovered	Recovered	Recovered	Recovered	Died 9th day	Died 9th day

Twenty-four patients were admitted with surface burns, three of whom were children (Table I). Intravenous fluid requirements were based on an assessment of the area burnt, using the rule of nines. A more accurate estimate was made later with the help of a pictorial chart.

Fluid replacement

Reconstituted plasma was used as colloid replacement, and a total of 110 pints was used. Patients with burns over 15% were infused, and the five most extensively burnt were given blood transfusions during the first 48 hours. One child with 6% partial-thickness burns needed intravenous rehydration as she became shocked 12 hours after the incident with a pyrexia of 37.8°C and a poor urinary output. Fluid requirements were calculated from the product of the patient's weight (kg) and the percentage of body surface burnt (% BSB) as the volume in millilitres of plasma required in the first 24 hours. Normal fluid requirements were given in addition either orally or intravenously. Oral fluids were encouraged from the start.

The regimen was kept under continuous review, and altered where necessary according to the following criteria:

(a) the clinical condition, based on nursing observations and frequent ward rounds. We found it helpful to conduct joint rounds with the pathologists and laboratory staff; (b) urine output, measured accurately from the start. In seven patients a urethral catheter was passed and the hourly output of urine recorded, providing a useful guide to the adequacy of fluid replacement; (c) laboratory findings—haemoglobin, packed cell volume (PCV), plasma proteins, and electrolytes were estimated in all patients. It was not feasible to estimate the haemoglobin and PCV more than twice daily even in severely burnt patients so we relied heavily on a combination of all criteria in assessing the fluid replacement; central venous pressure readings, which were taken on the three patients treated in the intensive care unit, were additionally helpful in these serious cases.

Though the initial assessment of the area burnt was almost invariably an overestimate there was only one case of overhydration. The tendency suggested by serial haemoglobin and PCV readings was of underhydration corrected over several days. There were no deaths during the first 48 hours though three patients became hypotensive and oliguric. They responded to more rapid infusion of plasma.

Antibiotic treatment

All patients were given tetanus vaccine and a course of antibiotics for five to seven days. Erythromycin, cloxacillin, or ampicillin were the initial drugs used. Gentamicin, carbenicillin, or cephaloridine were used in the most extensively burnt patients where indicated.

Isolation

Two wards of one- and four-bed units on the same floor as the theatre suite were used as a burns unit. These new wards had been in use for only three months, mainly for gynaecological cases, and there had been no cross-infection. A ratio of one nurse to each patient in the burns unit was maintained day and night. This was made possible by recruiting help from the list of retired and married trained nurses and the cancellation of all but emergency admissions to the hospital. One of the main operating theatres was used exclusively for all burns dressings.

Local care

Initially the burns were dressed with framycetin sulphate (Sofra-Tulle), but after 24 hours a supply of 1% silver sulphadiazine (Flamazine) was obtained and used for all subsequent dressings. Daily application gives the best results,[a] but this was not possible with the number of patients under treatment. Therefore most dressings were done on alternate days except where excessive soakage occurred, when they were done more frequently. After toilet of the burnt surface lengths of gauze on which a 3- to 5-mm layer of the cream had been smeared were applied. The gauze was covered with wool and held in place with crepe bandages or Netelast. General anaesthesia was used for dressings only in the children. All other patients were given a premedication of diazepam 10 mg intramuscularly, and further sedation with intravenous pethidine and diazepam was given in theatre under the supervision of an anaesthetist. With this regimen the patients tolerated the dressings well and had no pain on application of the cream.

Results

Of the 24 patients admitted with burns two died.

Case 4—A 54-year-old woman had 65% BSB, almost all full thickness. She also had a fractured pelvis, and her initial haematuria was attributed to this. A subsequent cystogram showed the bladder and urethra to be intact. She became anuric within 24 hours, after methaemoglobin and oxyhaemoglobin had been shown in the urine. There was no response to mannitol and frusemide. She became dyspnoeic on peritoneal dialysis, and after careful consideration, haemodialysis was started. A blood culture on the fourth day grew a non-haemolytic streptococcus, and she was treated with ampicillin and gentamicin. She died on the ninth day and was found at necropsy to have acute tubular necrosis with haemoglobin casts.

Case 5—This 35-year-old woman had 52% BSB, over half full thickness. The burned areas seemed clean, but a blood culture on the fourth day grew *Staphylococcus aureus*, which was treated with cephaloridine. The patient was fit for transfer to Scotland after 10 days, where her condition continued to fluctuate and she became increasingly catabolic. She died of bronchopneumonia on 30 September 1973, almost two months after the burn.

Morbidity

We were impressed by the absence of overt local infection, the usual yellow exudate being odourless and sterile. This accorded with the general well-being of the patients and the results of swabs which were taken from the burned surfaces. In extensive burns several swabs were taken from different areas of the body. Blood cultures were taken when septicaemia was suspected (Table II).

Table II—*Analysis of Positive Cultures from Burn Swabs. Results are Numbers of Cultures*

Days after burn:	0-3	4	5	6	7	8	9	10	11	12-28	Total
Non-haemolytic streptococcus	0	1*									1
Staphylococcus aureus	0	1*								5	6
Coliforms	0		2		2			1	2	2	9
Pseudomonas pyocyanea	0				1			2			3
Candida albicans					1						1

*Blood cultures.

Tests to show 'carry-over' of the antibacterial agent on to the culture medium[a] were negative, indicating that the high proportion of sterile swabs was a true index of the state of the burnt surfaces. There were 56 swabs which showed no growth. The positive coliform swabs were all taken from the buttocks or legs, and presumably resulted from faecal contamination of the burnt area. As silver sulphadiazine is maximally effective against Gram-negative organisms[b] we were surprised by the infrequency of *Staph. aureus*, particularly since the positive swabs were all taken from two patients between two and four weeks after the burn. During the second week the burnt surfaces became covered with a soft yellow adherent slough. Histological examination of this slough excised on the 25th day from one patient showed, 'a layer of necrotic connective tissue, lying upon a viable layer. The latter contains a few oedematous spaces with young capillaries, and a few lymphocytes. Surprising absence of inflammation.' The slough was slow to separate, presumably owing to the absence of proteinase-producing bacteria.[c] This may have caused a delay in skin grafting but was compensated by the reduction of infection.[d] The reports we had on the subsequent progress of these patients were favourable.

EMOTIONAL EFFECTS

In addition to two patients admitted primarily for emotional distress many others showed the effect of being involved in such a tragic incident. The effects included persistent vomiting, incontinence of urine, and mental withdrawal. Some patients were worrying about missing relatives, and two had lost their whole families. In spite of well-meaning attempts by relations to conceal the facts we felt it best to tell them the truth as soon as their condition permitted. With the sympathy and understanding of the nursing staff there were no major psychological crises during the period the patient were under our care.

Discussion

A major accident can occur at any time without warning, and prior thought and consultation between the emergency services involved is important. Rehearsal of such incidents are of limited value in our opinion, being expensive and disruptive of the normal routine and probably less useful than a regular discussion of the hospital emergency procedures and their publication among new members of staff. We had fortunately reviewed the emergency procedures some weeks earlier because of recent major alterations in the geography of the hospital which had made the previous regulations outdated.

The incident was unusual because of the large number of casualties and relatives who arrived at the hospital within 20 minutes of the warning being given. Though there was at first an element of chaos as the result of this large influx on the whole the casualties were dealt with in an efficient and humane manner. This is not to say that we were fully satisfied with our efforts, and were we to be presented with the same situation again we would pay particular attention to the following points.

Firstly, if circumstances permitted each casualty on arrival should be seen and assessed by a senior person to decide priority of treatment and then allocated to separate teams set up to deal with each type of case. Secondly, we found it useful and would certainly repeat the arrangement of allocating a nurse to each patient. This made for efficiency of communication, documentation, and treatment and also provided a large measure of comfort to each patient. Medical staff time was saved by the nurse writing brief notes at the dictation of the doctor. Finally we discovered the importance of adequate telephone lines to the hospital. There were no ex-directory lines and the switchboard was jammed rapidly by incoming inquiries. As a result essential outgoing calls to external staff and requests for extra supplies were held up. We feel that every hospital should have a number of ex-directory lines to cope with this sort of situation.

In treatment of major burns the first problem facing the non-specialist is that of fluid replacement. There are divergent views on both the volume and nature of the fluid to be used. Some regimens leave out colloid infusions altogether and emphasize the replacement of sodium and the correction of acidosis.[e] The diversity of opinions is confusing and we chose to stick to one regimen and modify it according to our basic knowledge of fluid replacement and the clinical state of the patients, which was assessed by frequent ward rounds. The management of the fluid requirements demands intensive care and we found that the time spent on ward rounds calculating fluid balance and adjusting the fluid regimen paid considerable dividends in the overall management of the patients. In most cases a urinary output greater than 2 litres a day was achieved and there were no serious biochemical disturbances.

In the local treatment of burns the application of antibacterial agents has been shown to have clear advantages in limiting infection.[a] Our experience with silver sulphadiazine has confirmed other reports of its effectiveness and lack of toxicity. After their transfer to other centres we had encouraging reports on the progress of the patients treated initially with silver sulphadiazine. We were particularly struck by the absence of infection and odour of the burns.

All three patients admitted with asphyxia had a relatively normal P_{CO_2} though they were deeply cyanosed. We were unfortunately unable to estimate P_{O_2} at the time of the disaster, but it can be assumed that it was very low in each case. A rising PCO_2, however, supported the clinical assessment of the need for IPPR. The Endotracheal intubation should be avoided unless indicated by the retention of secretions or the necessity for IPPR since it is particularly prone to produce tracheal ulceration in cases of asphyxia. There remains considerable controversy regarding the use of steroids in these patients. In our opinion the serious degree of bronchospasm that occurred made the use of steroids mandatory. We did not use them locally as an aerosol, but there is some evidence that this may be beneficial and perhaps avoid the need for systemic steroids.

We found diazepam carefully titrated by intravenous injection to be useful and safe for controlling restlessness, which can further aggravate respiratory distress. The use of carbenicillin by inhalation using an ultrasonic nebulizer as well as intravenously was very effective in the patient with pseudomonas infection.

We thank every member of the hospital staff and the many volunteers who worked so hard to help the victims of the disaster. We are also indebted to Miss A. Lees for preparation of the typescript.

References

[a] Fox, C. L. jun., *Annals of the New York Academy of Sciences*, 1968, **150**, 823.

[b] Fox, C. L., jun., *Archives of Surgery*, 1968, **96**, 184.

[c] Lowbury, E. J., *et al., Journal of Clinical Pathology*, 1962, **15**, 339.

[d] Lowbury, E. J., *et al., Lancet*, 1971, **2**, 1105.

[e] Settle, J. A. D., personal communication, 1973.

From: The *British Medical Journal*
24 May 1975, Vol. 2, p.407

Disaster planning—fact or fiction?

Since 1954 National Health Service hospitals have been required[a] to make arrangements for dealing with casualties resulting from a major accident, but unlike hospitals in the U.S.A. there has been no obligation for these plans to be tested to see if they actually work. Publications on disaster planning were already numerous [b–h] at the time of our last leading article,[i] and the eruption of urban guerilla warfare in the United

Kingdom has provided an opportunity of studying the plans of a number of hospitals in action.[j-l] Other disasters, including the Staines plane crash, the Summerland fire,[m] the Flixborough explosion, and the Moorgate train crash, have produced different problems in disaster management, but not one of them produced a new problem. Renewed interest in the practical aspects of disaster planning has been reflected in a number of seminars and conferences on the subject,[n o] but it seems that all the problems and techniques of disaster management have not as yet been appreciated, let alone put into practice, by those responsible in the hospital service and the community.

By definition, disaster occurs with little or no warning,[h] and casualties may start arriving at the hospital before the official alert has been given. Authority to initiate a hospital's disaster plan must be given to a doctor, nurse, or administrator actually in the hospital building at the time. Experience in Belfast confirms that adequate medical care in a disaster can often be provided by the on-duty medical and surgical teams, and that, by using a phased response, the alerting of medical, nursing, administrative, and ancillary staff can be adjusted to the nature of the disaster.[k] Hospital staff should be alerted by a detailed fan-out notification system to prevent the hospital switchboard from being overloaded with routine calls,[o] and staff should be allocated to their posts by the use of action cards kept on permanent display.[p q] Both the fan-out notification system and the action cards need to be tested regularly and relevant details of their role in the disaster plan should be explained to all new members of staff as part of their induction programme. The key to control of a sudden casualty load is a well-developed and tested casualty management plan. All casualties should be identified by a unique number and then undergo triage — sorting into categories of those needing urgent and non-urgent treatment, and those that are dead. Standard hospital documentation should be used wherever possible. One of the basic fundamentals of disaster planning is that wherever possible individuals should perform familiar tasks with familiar equipment in familiar places.

The concept of the one 'designated' hospital enshrined in H.M.(54)51 remains a stumbling block to present-day disaster planning on a district, area, or regional basis. Spreading the casualty load in distance and time to a number of casualty receiving hospitals is the key to preventing one particular hospital from being swamped with casualties, and responsibility for this rests ultimately with the ambulance service. The ambulance service remains the Cinderella of the emergency services in both status and finance, but it is becoming increasingly recognized that the ambulance man has a vital part to play in primary medical care. The number of areas with advanced training schemes for ambulance men is increasing, and the division of the service into two tiers with separation of the patient-care from the transport function cannot long be delayed. Experienced medical staff are important at the scene of an accident or disaster, but a well trained, equipped, and organized ambulance service can relieve the hospital service of providing a team of doctors and nurses just at the time when their skills are most needed in the hospital.

Control of nearly every disaster fails because of inadequate communication and co-ordination at all levels of every emergency service. With modern radiotelephonic techniques it is possible to connect a radio link into a telephone switchboard, and the provision of this means of communication between every casualty receiving hospital and ambulance control is long overdue.

There are still many difficulties in disaster planning, and the ultimate responsibility for maintaining the readiness of hospital and community plans, both local and national, remains unresolved. Hospitals in the United Kingdom are ill-prepared to deal with disasters. This needs knowledge, will, and money. The knowledge is already available.

References

[a] Ministry of Health, *Medical Arrangements for Dealing with Major Accidents* H.M.(54)51. London, H.M.S.O., 1954.

[b] American Hospital Association, *Principles of Disaster Preparedness for Hospitals.* Chicago, American Hospital Association, 1971.

[c] American Hospital Association, *Readings in Disaster Planning for Hospitals.* Chicago, American Hospital Association, 1966.

[d] Garb, S., and Eng., E., *Disaster Handbook*, 2nd edn. New York, Springer, 1969.

[e] Magruder, D. M., *Hospital Management*, 1968, **105**, 79.

[f] Miller, P. J., *Injury*, 1971, **2**, 168.

[g] Savage, P. E. A., *Injury*, 1971, **3**, 49.

[h] Thorpe, G. L., *Hospital Progress*, 1965, **46**, 115.

[i] *British Medical Journal*, 1972, **3**, 3.

[j] Caro, D., and Irving, M., *Lancet*, 1973, **1**, 1433.

[k] Rutherford, W. H., *Injury*, 1973, **4**, 189.

[l] Rutherford, W. H., *British Medical Journal*, 1975, **1**, 443.

[m] Hart, R. J., *et al.*, *British Medical Journal*, 1975, **1**, 256.

[n] Sillar, W. (ed), *A Guide to Disaster Management*. Glasgow, Action for Disaster, 1974.

[o] Richardson, J. W. (ed), *Disaster Planning Symposium*, Haslar, 1974. Bristol, Wright, 1975

[p] Savage, P. E. A., *British Medical Journal*, 1972, **3**, 42.

[q] Hirst, W., and Savage, P. E. A., *Nursing Times*, 1974, **70**, 186.

[r] Snook, R., *Medical Aid at Accidents*. London, Update Publications, 1975.

From: The *British Medical Journal*
2 August 1975, Vol. 3, pp.287-289

Surgery of violence
the Tower of London bomb explosion
Keith Tucker, Alan Lettin

After the detonation of a bomb in the Tower of London 37 people were brought to St. Bartholomew's Hospital. The explosion caused numerous severe injuries of a type rarely seen in peacetime.

Introduction

During the past few years St. Bartholomew's Hospital, situated within the City of London, has received many civilian casualties resulting from letter bombs, a car bomb, and more recently from the explosion of what was probably a 'carrier bag' bomb detonated inside the Tower of London. This has presented unfamiliar problems for the rescue services, the accident and emergency department, and the individual doctor.

Each of these explosions has produced its own pattern of injuries. The Old Bailey car bomb caused 160 casualties, most of whose injuries were caused by flying glass and metal and not directly by the blast, which was easily dissipated in the open air. On that occasion 19 patients were admitted to hospital, but only four had severe injuries.[a] The explosion within the confines of the Tower of London injured fewer people, but these injuries were generally more severe. This bomb contained 10 lb (4.5 kg) of explosive and it had been placed alongside the wooden carriage of a 50 cwt (2500 kg) 18th century bronze cannon in the armoury of the White Tower. The room, which measured 68 ft (21 m) long 28 ft (8.5 m) wide and 20 ft (6 m) high, had stone walls 15 ft (4.5 m) thick. The casualties were grouped around the cannon, and their injuries were caused by 'blast', fragments of wood, stone, and metal or by being thrown against the floor and walls. The gun carriage was destroyed and the cannon thrown to the floor.

Thirty-seven people were injured and 19 required admission to hospital; of these, 10 (27%) had severe multiple injuries. One patient died. The injuries and the numbers of patients sustaining them were as follows: Fractured skull 2, injuries to the facial skeleton 2, fractures of other bones 10, abdominal injuries 2, lung injuries 2, injuries to skin and integument 20, burns 10, eye injuries 4, ear injuries 22.

Organization

The first casualties arrived at the hospital within 20 minutes of the explosion through a traffic-free clearway established by the police. On arrival previously prepared and similarly numbered emergency record cards, pathology and X-ray request forms, and observation charts were attached to each patient with an identification bracelet.

As soon as the magnitude of the disaster became apparent all available medical, nursing, and ancillary staff were summoned to the receiving area. Sufficient medical staff were available to allow one doctor to devote his whole attention to the examination and documentation of a single patient, initiating resuscitation, antibiotic therapy, and antitetanus prophylaxis. This initial assessment was complicated by the fact that many of the patients had been deafened and some spoke no English.

A consultant general surgeon and a consultant orthopaedic surgeon, guided by this initial assessment, reviewed each patient and determined further treatment. Anaesthetists were on hand to help with respiratory and major resuscitation problems, and a pathologist was present in the receiving area organizing supplies of blood for transfusion.

Though a mobile medical team was dispatched to the Tower, as in the Old Bailey incident, its presence was superfluous. The injured had not been trapped, and there were sufficient ambulances to transfer them all to hospital without the need for any preliminary assessment of treatment.

Seven fully staffed main operating theatres were available within one hour of the first casualties arriving at the hospital, four by curtailing operating lists already in progress. This relieved the surgeons in charge of the difficult task of establishing any degree of priority in the treatment of the seven most severely injured patients. In the operating theatres these patients came under an appropriate surgical team headed by a consultant, senior registrar, or registrar. Two consultant plastic surgeons, a consultant neurosurgeon, and a consultant faciomaxillary surgeon were incorporated in the teams requiring their specialist skills. Further resuscitation and assessment of each patient took place in the relative calm of the anaesthetic room before and after induction of anaesthesia. Most of the X-ray films which were required were taken at this stage. The consultants in charge visited each operating theatre after their initial duties in the emergency department were completed to advise on policy and co-ordinate the overall management. All patients had been transferred from the receiving area within two hours of the first arrival.

Inquiries from the police, the press, the public, and relatives were dealt with by the senior administrative staff, as recommended by Caro and Irving.[a]

Treatment

The immediate surgical treatment was restricted to repairing vital organs and wound toilet. This was accomplished in nearly all patients within 12 hours of the explosion. One patient was observed overnight for signs of visceral damage before his simple wounds were attended to. Initial antibiotic therapy, consisting of penicillin to combat potential clostridial infections and an antibiotic effective against a broad spectrum of other organisms, was continued until wounds had healed.

OPEN WOUNDS

Seventeen patients had multiple extensive contaminated wounds containing wood, splinters, stone, metal, and clothing. The larger wounds were obvious but often it was not until the superficial debris had been gently removed with a scrubbing brush that smaller penetrating wounds were found. The classical treatment for wounds of this nature was followed.

After liberal cleansing with Savlon (cetrimide) all flayed skin and the wound edges were excised down to the deep fascia. Contaminated and devitalized fat, fascia, and muscle were removed to expose healthy tissues. Small areas of discolouration remaining on the skin after the initial 'scrubbing' were often the entry wounds of surprisingly large pieces of debris, and these were carefully treated in the same way. Some 300 small pieces of wood were removed from one patient alone.

All but five wounds, including an amputation, were left open for later closure. The dorsum of a hand which had been degloved was partially covered with Thiersch grafts. A clean incised facial wound, a compound comminuted fracture of the skull sustained in falling, and a contaminated leg wound were sutured, the latter under local anaesthetic. It is significant that this leg wound subsequently became infected and broke down before healing by granulation.

All the wounds were inspected under general anaesthetic between the fifth and seventh days after the incident. Most were clean and suitable for closure, but in addition seven patients required multiple Thiersch grafts. The amputation was closed with drainage.

The severe blast injuries of both calves sustained by one patient were heavily infected and necrotic, resulting in septicaemia and renal failure. Further exploration disclosed more debris and a more extensive debridement was carried out, which resulted in immediate improvement of the patient's condition. Two weeks later the wounds were grafted, but healing eventually occurred by granulation. With the exception of this patient and three other local infections all wounds had healed within three weeks of the explosion. The infection was predominantly *Pseudomonas aeruginora* (*pyocyanea*), and this was eradicated by topical application of acetic acid and exposure to a current of hot air from a hair dryer.

BURNS

Ten patients suffered flash burns to areas of uncovered skin. These were treated by exposure unless adjacent to open wounds. All healed without scarring, though two patients required plasma infusions more in keeping with full thickness loss. Burning clothing in two patients resulted in minor full thickness burns, for which grafting was unnecessary.

INTRA-ABDOMINAL INJURIES

Two children suffered intra-abdominal injuries. One was caused by a sliver of wood 18 in (45 cm) long penetrating the left flank and entering the cortex of the left kidney. The wood was removed, the kidney preserved, and the wound closed by delayed primary suture. The other child sustained a 'closed' laceration of the left lobe of the liver. This was not suspected until three hours after the explosion. The laceration was sutured.

INJURIES TO CRANIUM AND FACIAL SKELETON

One patient sustained severe damage to the frontal lobes and brain stem associated with multiple compound facial fractures and a compound comminuted fracture of the skull. After intubation and transfusion a tracheostomy was performed, but before her injuries could be treated she died.

An 11-year-old boy sustained a compound comminuted fracture of the occipital and parietal bones when he was blown over. This injury was associated with cortical blindness and minor concussion, but it did not involve damage to the dura or venous sinuses. Immediate debridement and skin closure were performed. One week later the remaining fragments of bone were removed, and three months later the defect was closed with a tantalum plate. The cortical blindness has almost completely recovered.

A boy of 13 sustained a comminuted fracture of the mandible and maxillae. He also had facial burns and a few small lacerations. On the day of the incident the jaw was stabilized with wire and an airway maintained via a nasopharyngeal tube.

FRACTURES

There were 20 fractures of bones other than the skull and facial skeleton in ten patients. Except for an open fracture of the pubis the fractures were all confined to limb bones, and 10 were compound.

The fractures were initially treated conservatively with the exception of a fractured tibia and fibula associated with such severe vascular, nerve, and soft tissue damage that an amputation 3½ in (9 cm) below the knee joint had to be performed. Subsequent internal fixation was necessary in three patients. A very unstable simple supracondylar fracture of the humerus associated with a radial nerve palsy was treated by open reduction and internal fixation three weeks after the incident. The radial nerve palsy has partially recovered, but unfortunately myositis ossificans has developed.

A compound fracture of the right tibia and fibula with extensive anterior skin loss which required Thiersch grafts was the only fracture showing no evidence of union at 10 weeks. After the skin had completely healed this was plated and grafted with autogenous cancellous bone through a posterior approach.

One boy had a severely mutilated hand in which there were compound fractures of the three ulnar metacarpals and fractures of the little and ring fingers. The little finger was amputated on the day of the incident. A week later the wound was sufficiently clean for the metacarpal fractures to be stabilized with Kirschner wires and the hand to be covered with a pedicle graft from the anterior abdominal wall.

JOINTS

Two patients sustained open injuries to the ankle joint. In both patients the joint was initially cleaned, the capsule closed, and the overlying skin left open. Neither joint became infected.

LUNGS

Chest X-ray films showed evidence of contusion of the lower lobes of the right lung in two children. Fortunately neither patient developed 'blast lung syndrome', and from this standpoint their clinical condition was always satisfactory. Serial X-ray films have shown that the changes have resolved. No other chest injuries were detected.

EAR INJURIES

Twenty-two patients with ear injuries suffered deafness, tinnitus, pain, and bleeding from the external meatus. There were 16 perforated ear drums in 12 patients. Audiograms showed varying degrees of sensorineural damage in 21 patients.

The initial treatment was always conservative. Local treatment was prohibited unless there were large pieces of debris in the meatus. The patients were instructed not to allow their ears to get wet. Eight perforated drums healed spontaneously, and four myringoplasties have so far been performed, of which three were successful. Serial audiograms have shown varying degrees of recovery in those patients with sensorineural damage, but in only two (both children) has recovery been complete. One patient complained of total deafness, for which no organic cause could be found, and his hearing suddenly returned spontaneously a few days after the explosion. No damage to the inner ear causing leakage of fluid from the cochlea was detected.

EYE INJURIES

Four patients received eye injuries which would have necessitated hospital admission in their own right. One boy suffered a laceration of the left cornea, which required suturing, and multiple intraocular and intracorneal foreign bodies were detected in the right eye (probably cordite). The sight in the left eye is now satisfactory, but the right eye will be permanently damaged, and the right lens has been removed for post-traumatic cataract. Three patients had corneal abrasions, which responded rapidly to traditional conservative therapy.

MENTAL ILLNESS

Only four patients complained of psychiatric symptoms. For three weeks one woman experienced a severe exacerbation of her previous depression and anxiety neurosis. Another patient had similar milder symptoms. One man suffered from recurrent nightmares and agoraphobia on leaving hospital three months after the explosion. Another patient, referred to above, suffered from hysterical deafness.

These symptoms all improved with reassurance and tranquillizers.

FURTHER FOLLOW-UP

In all, 47 surgical procedures were undertaken on the day of the explosion and over subsequent weeks. Eight patients were in hospital for more than three months.

Follow-up is by no means complete, and it is hoped that further recovery will take place in those patients who still have symptoms. Many patients have returned to their own countries and further assessment of results is difficult.

Conclusions

The multiplicity and variety of injuries caused by an explosion may be considerable. Many doctors, nurses, and ancillary staff with the specialist skills of a large hospital are required to give adequate treatment to so many patients simultaneously. These skills and facilities are not readily available in every hospital, and this should be considered by the rescue services when they are evacuating a disaster area. A traffic-free route can usually be created through the most crowded streets to a major hospital by the police.

The initial assessment of each patient can be difficult and time-consuming, and preferably should not be carried out at the site of the explosion. Mobile teams are required only when casualties are trapped or where transport facilities are limited, delaying transfer to hospital. We agree with Boyd[c] that rapid evacuation of casualties to a large centre without any form of immediate treatment is to be preferred.

The classical precepts of radical debridement and delayed primary or secondary suture must be rigorously adhered to in the treatment of open wounds if complications are to be avoided. The frequency of serious ear and eye injuries after an explosion makes it imperative that the injured are all examined by an ophthalmologist and ear specialist at the earliest opportunity.

We are indebted to the members of the consultant staff of the hospital under whose care the casualties were admitted and to those others who treated them for their permission to publish their article. We are particularly grateful to Messrs. M. A. Bedford, R. J. McNab Jones, and

D. Winstock, who advised us on the details and management of the injuries peculiar to their respective specialties.

References

a Caro, D., and Irving, M., *Lancet*, 1973, **1**, 1433.
b Edwards, H. C., *Recent Advances in Surgery*, 3rd edn., p.3. London, Churchill, 1948.
c Boyd, N. A., *Annals of the Royal College of Surgeons of England*, 1975, **56**, 15.

ANNEX 4

Method of calculation
of casualty numbers

1. Some data for the population distribution over the area in question are required. These are usually taken from census figures.

2. The selected targets are located on the ground, and the explosive yields and heights of burst of bombs are decided.

Burns caused by direct thermal radiation
(if these are estimated)

3. A series of concentric rings is drawn for each bomb, centred on the point immediately below the explosion or 'ground zero', whose radii represent the ranges of selected levels of thermal radiant exposure. These radii are calculated from the yields and burst heights specified in step 2, allowing also for some assumptions about atmospheric visibility.

4. Assumptions are made about the percentage of the population who are exposed in direct line of sight to the fireball. Burns casualties are then calculated using a series of values which give the degree of burning, and the resulting deaths and injuries, for the selected ranges of exposure level.

The numbers killed by burns are subtracted from the initial population, and the numbers of injured and survivors noted.

Blast casualties

5. A second series of concentric rings is drawn for each bomb, to represent selected peak overpressure contours. The radii of those circles are again calculated directly from the yields and heights of burst specified in step 2.

6. The total population falling within each of these rings is counted, and casualties are calculated for blast using a series of values which give percentages killed and injured in the selected peak overpressure ranges.

The numbers killed by blast are subtracted from the surviving population, and the numbers of injured (from either burns or blast) and uninjured survivors noted. The assumption may be made that those suffering a combination of blast and burns injuries will die, in which case their numbers are also removed from the survivors.

Fall-out casualties

7. Ground-burst bombs only are considered; and some assumptions are made about those physical characteristics of the weapons which determine the nature of the radioactive products of explosion.

8. Assumptions are made about the prevailing wind speed and direction.

9. For each bomb, a series of ellipses is constructed which in every case have one focus at 'ground zero' and the major axis aligned with the wind direction. These ellipses mark radiation dose rate contours. They are highly idealised representations of the pattern in which fall-out would actually be deposited. Each ellipse corresponds to some specified rate at which a person would receive a radiation dose at that range, at a given time after the explosion. The lengths of the ellipses down-wind (and so the areas of the ellipses) are directly dependent on the assumed wind speed.

10. For every affected point or zone on the ground, two values of the dose rate are found: first at the time when the moving radioactive cloud arrives, and second at the end of some arbitrarily chosen time period when radiation levels have substantially reduced (very often a limit of two weeks is taken). The radiation dose accumulated (by persons in the open) during this interval is calculated.

The computation is somewhat complex, and is divided into two parts: the period in which the radioactive cloud is passing overhead ('time of arrival' to 'time of completion' of fall-out); and the period after the cloud has passed. Allowances must be made for the accumulation of the fall-out on the ground in the first period, and the radioactive decay of the fall-out throughout both periods.

11. Steps 7 to 10 give theoretical values for the doses which would be received assuming an absolutely flat ground surface. These are multiplied by a factor to allow for the roughness of the terrain (usually 0.7 for relatively flat land, and 0.5 for hilly districts).

12. For zones where fall-out is received from more than one bomb, the accumulated doses from each are summed together.

13. These accumulated doses relate to persons exposed in the open. They are reduced by a 'protective factor' or PF for those persons

assumed to be inside houses or shelters. The value of the protective factor depends on consideration of the form and materials of construction of the shelter; on assumptions (in relation to houses and flats) as to whether the occupants have taken any special precautions such as blocking windows and doors or building 'inner refuges'; and on assumptions about the proportion of time, during the period of risk, that the occupants actually spend inside. In some cases a range or 'spectrum' of protective factors is taken, to represent different sheltering conditions.

14. Fall-out casualties are calculated for each zone depending on the dose received, using some chosen dose/injury model. This is usually in the form of an S-shaped curve, giving the percentage of the exposed population who would die at differing dose values. A second curve may be used to give percentages seriously ill with radiation sickness. Again there may be assumptions made that those suffering some combination of radiation sickness with other injuries, will die.

Final totals of survivors, and dead and injured from all three causes, can then be drawn up.

Commentary

It is possible, indeed very probable, that people might be injured from more than one cause. Thus among those counted as injured from blast there may be some subsequently counted as injured also by burns. The same applies for both kinds of injury and serious radiation sickness. In some studies assumptions are made about such combinations of injuries and whether they are likely to result in death. This probability of death from multiple injury may well be higher than would be arrived at by considering the independent effects to be simply additive. (The injuries are said to be 'synergistic'.) Thus one effect of radiation sickness is to lower the body's resistance to infection, and in these conditions mechanical injuries and burns would be much more dangerous.

Since the range of damage and physical effects of modern nuclear weapons is so great, it is further possible that individuals might receive the same general class of injury from more than one bomb. There is the additional complication that several bombs might fall in the same area, but separate in time. It is almost impossible to predict what the cumulative consequences might be for casualties. Extraordinarily, there were even a few individuals unfortunate or fortunate enough to be in Hiroshima on 6 August 1945, who travelled to Nagasaki for the 9 August, and survived both bombings.

Emergencies at nuclear reactor plants

The Generating Board's Safety Departments have a responsibility for monitoring and assessing independently the safety of plant; in addition, plant has to be operated in accordance with the site licence issued by the Nuclear Installations Inspectorate on behalf of the Health and Safety Executive. Nevertheless, as a precaution, each station has an emergency plan for dealing with any accident that might affect the public or the surrounding environment. The plan includes arrangements for a temporary ban on foodstuffs produced locally and for the temporary evacuation of people in any 30% sector within about two-thirds of a mile downwind from the station. It is also a siting requirement that this distance could be extended to about two miles without presenting the police with any undue problems.

Implementation of an emergency plan

The County Police and the Local Authority cooperate in the production of a comprehensive emergency plan for the police, fire, ambulance and welfare services. These include the evacuation of people and the provisions of reception centres with temporary sleeping accommodation and canteen facilities. Any evacuation required during a nuclear emergency would be carried out in accordance with these plans, and no special arrangements are required.

The Emergency Controller would inform the police of any emergency and the police would act as the channel of communication with senior officials of the other emergency services and of the County Council. Direct request for assistance from local fire brigade or ambulance services might also be made by the Emergency Controller.

The police would set up a communications centre near the power station's Emergency Control Centre and, if necessary, take steps to prevent access to affected areas near the site.

Transport of Fuel

Emergency arrangements for the transport of fuel

An accident during transit would not lead to releases of large quantities of radioactivity because of the care taken in the design, manufacture and testing of the transport flasks. Nevertheless, arrangements exist that enable assistance to be brought in for any situation. These arrangements involve not only the Generating Boards but also British Rail, fire brigades, police forces and emergency services.

Road transport for radioactive material excluding nuclear fuel

Should an accident occur during transport by road and radiological assistance be required, the police will institute arrangements made under the NAIR scheme. NAIR stands for National Arrangements for Incidents involving Radioactivity, and is the system by means of which assistance may be obtained to deal with accidents involving packages of radioactive material. On being informed of any such emergency, the police will initiate whatever action is necessary to summon quickly specialist advice on how to deal with any radiological hazards that may arise during transport operations. There are two stages of assistance, the first (Stage 1) generally being provided by physicists from local hospitals and the second (Stage 2) by the United Kingdom Atomic Energy Authority, the CEGB, the SSEB, British Nuclear Fuels Ltd, the Radiochemical Centre Ltd, the Ministry of Defence or the National Radiological Protection Board.

Road transport of irradiated fuel

The Generating Boards' Fuel Transport Flask Emergency Plan contains arrangements made to cover the road transport of fuel flasks between a power station and its railhead.

Should an accident occur, the road-transporter crew will immediately notify the power station concerned and will remain with the vehicle until help arrives to ensure that members of the public are kept at a safe distance. A Co-ordinating Officer at the power station will call out the Flask Emergency Team and will notify the local police, Board Headquarters and, if necessary, the fire brigade, local authorities and certain Government Departments.

Rail transport

In conjunction with British Rail, the Generating Boards operate a contingency plan that supplements and is similar to the NAIR scheme. In the event of an accident, actions under the plan are initiated by British Rail, who inform the police, fire brigade and a specified officer at either CEGB's National Control or, in Scotland, SSEB's Hunterston power station. A team of experts is dispatched to the scene of the accident, and the police and the fire brigade acting on telephone advice from National Control or the power station take the necessary steps to protect the public.

To cover any possible emergency, the whole of England, Scotland and Wales is divided into areas in which organisations such as nuclear power stations and atomic energy establishments are located. These possess teams of highly qualified staff who are specially trained and equipped to deal with emergencies. In addition, the emergency establishments provide extensive back-up in terms of facilities and manpower. The response and performance of the emergency teams are regularly tested.

Home Defence Circular HDC (77)1: The preparation and organisation of The Health Service for war

Summary

This circular deals with the organisation for war of the Health Service in England; the introduction of an emergency system of control, and cancels previous Civil Defence memorandum.

Introduction

1. Existing plans for the Health Service in war are based on the HM(CD) series of memoranda issued by the Ministry of Health. Since 1968 however successive governments have introduced modifications to home defence policies and these, together with the re-organisation of the National Health Service, have rendered obsolete the plans prepared by the former Regional Hospital Boards. The HM(CD) memoranda are therefore cancelled and this circular, which is the first of a new series, explains the basis on which the Health Service is now to be prepared and organised for war.

2. The Home Office co-ordinates the issue of guidance by central government departments about home defence matters and has issued memoranda (under the ES series of circulars) on home defence planning, to local and other public authorities. Copies of memoranda relevant to the Health Service have been sent to all Health Authorities and copies of this and subsequent circulars will be sent to local and public authorities as appropriate. This circular should be read in conjunction with the Home Office memoranda and attention is drawn particularly to:

Home Defence Boundaries (ES1/1973)
Home Defence Planning Assumptions (ES3/1973)
Machinery of Government in War (ES7/1973)
Survival Under Fall-out Conditions (ES10/1974)

3. The issue of Home Defence planning circulars and of this circular, does not mean that the Government consider that war is imminent or inevitable. It is however only prudent to take reasonable precautions to mitigate the effects of a possible attack and so to plan the organisation and control of the Health Service that it may be able to make an effective contribution to the subsequent recovery of the country. The purpose of this circular is therefore to set out the preparations that Health authorities should now make and the organisation they would adopt, to meet the effects of any major attack on this country. Further circulars will be issued from time to time to deal with particular aspects of preparation for war and the action to be taken after attack.

Planning assumptions

4. Home Defence Planning Assumptions (ES3/73) differ from the previous Civil Defence policy and certain features of the new policy have a particular bearing on Health Service planning. Health Service plans should therefore be made on the following assumptions:

a. The general aim in a crisis would be to keep disruption of the social, economic and industrial life of the country to a minimum as long as possible. Any large scale re-organisation of the Health Service, to put it on a war footing, should therefore be avoided.

b. No part of the country could expect to avoid the effects of an attack. Those areas not directly attacked might suffer from radioactive fall-out; would certainly feel the effects of the destruction and disruption elsewhere of supplies, services and transport and might receive an influx of refugees. All Health Authorities must therefore plan to meet the consequences of an attack on any part of the country.

c. The pattern of attack and radioactive fall-out cannot be accurately predicted. The public would be better protected by remaining in their own homes than by moving to other areas where the local and other public authorities might well be unable to provide shelter, food or essential services. The Government do not propose to arrange for any official evacuation of the public and, through press, television and radio, would advise against random movement.

d. Fall-out conditions are likely to impose severe restraints on movement after an attack, possibly for several days. Immediate medical care for survivors might not therefore be possible and medical staff, who would be irreplaceable except in the long term, should not be wasted by allowing them to enter highly radioactive areas to assist casualties.

General considerations

5. It is possible that a future war might begin with a period of non-nuclear conventional war and small scale attacks against vital installations or centres of Government could not be discounted. It is unlikely however that conventional war on this scale could continue for long without either a settlement of the international dispute or a sudden escalation into nuclear war.

6. A nuclear strike would give rise to radioactive fall-out. The spread and intensity of the fall-out would depend upon many factors at the time, but it may be assumed that the greater part of the country would be covered, in varying degrees, by plumes of highly radioactive dust, in many cases overlapping. The intensity of this fall-out would prevent, in most areas, any outside movement during at least the first 48 hours after an attack and, in any case, the whole of the United Kingdom would be under a RED Warning against the possibility of further attacks during this period. For the first 48 hours after an attack therefore, little or no life-saving activity would be possible, except on the most limited self help basis.

7. Radiation decays very rapidly in the first few hours and days after a strike, but thereafter decay is slow. An initial level of 1000 rph may fall to 10 rph in 48 hours, but would not reach 1 rph for 14 days. Some people would receive an immediate radiation dose from the explosion but most would receive doses from the subsequent fall-out, the amount depending in part on the protective factor of their accommodation. Further exposure in the open to radiation would have serious and probably lethal effect until the ambient rate had fallen to 0.5 rph. When the dose rate had fallen to 4 rph however release from cover could be allowed for 1 hour in 24 and further release periods could be extended as radiation levels decline. General life saving operations in areas of fall-out might not be possible therefore until days or even weeks after a nuclear strike.

8. Certain built up areas may be regarded as potential targets but there are many possible targets in rural areas. No part of the country can therefore be assumed to be safe both from attack and from radioactive fall-out from attacks elsewhere. Nevertheless, if the total destruction or isolation of health service resources is to be avoided, some redeployment of medical and nursing staff, medical supplies, ambulances and equipment would be essential. The major concentration of hospitals lies in the centres of large towns and cities and contains a high proportion of the most skilled staff and essential medical supplies and equipment, while a high proportion of patients attending those

hospitals comes from the periphery of the urban areas. The redeployment of resources could reduce the possibility of total destruction and bring them closer to those who would have most need of them after an attack. As a pre-condition to redeployment, all patients medically and socially fit to be sent home would have to be discharged and hospitals would have to accept emergency cases only.

9. The peacetime administrative structure of the Health Service is unsuited to the needs of war, when a clear system of control would be needed for the rapid acquisition and redevelopment of surviving resources. A control structure would be required which could be activated before an attack and which would relate to the various levels of wartime regional government.

10. The regions and sub-regions adopted for Government control (ES1/73) and the boundaries of local authority counties and districts do not, in many cases, match the Health Service organisation and where they do, they match at different levels in the non-metropolitan and the metropolitan countries. It would be undesirable however, in a period of crisis, to add to the burdens of the Health Service by altering the administrative boundaries. It is not intended therefore to alter boundaries or agency arrangements before an attack, but to relate the health service structure to the regional government organisation as well as the present relationship of boundaries allows. Whatever the boundary arrangements, adjustment might well be needed after an attack. Where discrepancies between local government and health authorities lead to practical problems before then they will no doubt be the subject of local consultation between the authorities concerned.

11. After an attack, the number of casualties might be quite beyond the resources of existing health services. Hospitals might be destroyed or isolated and the care of casualties might have to be undertaken largely by volunteers working in the community under professional supervision. Whenever possible however the aim should be to base the care of casualties on surviving and expanded hospitals, so as to simplify the re-establishment of control and the distribution of supplies; to provide centres for the medical care of serious cases; to create a firm base from which the remaining staff could work and to raise morale of both public and staff by demonstrating a determination to re-build the Health Service, albeit in a modified form.

Aims

12. The aims of the Health Service will be to provide medical and nursing care for the casualties of war and the sick and to maintain a basis for future reconstruction.

Layout of the circular

13. The circular is in four Parts:

Part I (Preparation for War) sets out the measures that Health Authorities may be required to take during a period of crisis, to prepare the Health Service to meet the effects of war;

Part II (Organisation in War) deals with the transition from the peace-time system of administration to a war-time system of control;

Part III (Casualty Policy) outlines procedures for the care of casualties after a major attack;

Part IV (Summary of Action) lists the action that Health Authorities should now take.

PART I—PREPARATION FOR WAR

14. It is assumed (ES3/1973) that there would be three to four weeks political warning of the outbreak of war, but Health Authorities must be prepared to complete essential action within a much shorter period. The aim of the preparations would be to reduce the hospital population as far as possible, to provide space for the care of casualties, and to disperse staff, essential supplies and equipment, to reduce the risk of the total destruction of resources. Health Authorities including Boards of Governors should now plan for these measures; implementation would be authorised by the Secretary of State, when circumstances required.

Discharge of patients

15. During a period of crisis and when so directed, Health Authorities should arrange for all patients in hospitals, nursing and convalescent homes, whose retention was not medically essential, to be sent home. The purpose of this evacuation would be to free hospitals to deal with later casualties, to afford patients the greater protection that dispersal to their own homes would provide and to allow for the redistribution of equipment and staff. It is hoped that there would be sufficient warning of an attack to allow seven days for the discharge of patients, but plans should allow for a more rapid discharge should this become necessary.

16. The selection of patients for discharge should be made on medical grounds and on the availability of home accommodation and care. For the latter, the advice of the local authority social services department would in some cases be needed and arrangements should be made with

local authorities to provide the maximum effort to check home conditions. Discharge should not however be held up merely because home conditions were not ideal or could not be checked and it must be accepted that the crisis would entail hardship. Criteria for selecting patients for discharge should be based on those which would have to be adopted, following an attack with many casualties, for the selection of patients for hospital treatment. Consultants would therefore need to consider whether, after an attack, they would expect to retain or discharge a patient in the same clinical condition as those under review. The numbers to be discharged cannot be pre-determined and in some cases, for example, geriatrics, no discharges might be possible; it might be expected however that the number of patients to be discharged would be of the following order, although it is stressed that these figures should in no way be taken as targets to be fulfilled;

Maternity cases	70%
Convalescents	100%
Acute cases	60%
Sick children	70%
Non active infections and chest cases	50%
Psychiatric cases	15%

The policy for the discharge of patients would also apply to the nursing and convalescent homes with contractual arrangements with an AHA and, at the discretion of the Health Authority, to private hospitals and nursing homes (Paragraph 26).

17. Arrangements should be made for the transport of patients to their homes using where necessary ambulances, the hospital car service and hired vehicles. The remaining patients should be redistributed within the hospital or home to make the maximum use of the protective factors in the building, and the establishment should be prepared for a situation in which radioactivity prevented any movement outside and all public utilities were out of action. At least 14 days of essential foods and 16 litres of water per person, should be stored during the warning period and kept topped up and, following an attack, strict rationing should be introduced.

18. Hospitals should continue to accept emergency cases during a period of crisis but out-patient clinics should be closed. Diagnostic pathology and X-ray services should continue on an emergency basis. Any cases admitted should be discharged as soon as their clinical condition permitted.

Dispersal of medical supplies and equipment

19. A high proportion of the medical supplies and equipment most needed after an attack is concentrated in hospitals situated in urban areas. A single attack could therefore destroy the greater part of a Health Authority's resources or could render them temporarily inaccessible because of radioactivity or the blocking of roads. AHAs should therefore prepare to disperse, as widely as possible within their Area, those drugs (and the means of administering them), anaesthetic equipment, dressings, surgical instruments and portable items of medical equipment, essential to the treatment of casualties. Arrangements should be made to disperse these priority items in balanced packs to hospitals, nursing homes and other health service establishment, to provide as wide a dispersion as possible. Where the greater part of an AHA lies within a built up area, the dispersal arrangements should be made on a Regional basis. Plans should also be made to disperse any home defence stores held by RHAs, and arrangements would be made to issue to RHAs any such stores held centrally.

Blood transfusion service

20. Blood and certain blood products are essential for the proper care of casualties. RHAs should arrange for the dispersal of stocks of such blood as may be available in Regional Transfusion Centres and earmark refrigerators (preferably with independent generators) in advance. As much plasma volume expander (dried plasma, plasma protein fraction, or plasma substitute) as possible should also be dispersed. After an attack great reliance would have initially to be placed on local blood collection and stocks of appropriate equipment and blood grouping reagents should also be dispersed. Premises for re-establishing the RTC, should the need arise, should be earmarked.

Ambulance services

21. The scope for the further dispersal of the ambulance service may be small, but the appropriate Health Authorities should prepare plans to leave in operation, before an attack, sufficient ambulances to support an emergency service only and to disperse the remainder. In the case of London, South West Thames RHA should prepare a plan, in conjunction with the other Thames RHAs, for the whole GLC area.

22. Ambulances should be dispersed so as to provide an emergency wireless network between all the Health Service headquarters and

hospitals within the Region or Area. While Ambulance Service wireless installations would be vulnerable to the effects of nuclear strike, any communications remaining after an attack would be a valuable aid to the exercise of control and the collection of information.

Dispersal of staff

23. The same considerations that apply to the safety of patients and equipment apply equally to staff. A large proportion of Health Service staff are concentrated in central urban areas which could become isolated in the event of attack. Trained staff are the most valuable asset possessed by the Health Service and could be replaced only in the very long term. As soon as patients have been sent home therefore all staff not required to operate an emergency service should themselves be sent home or dispersed within the Area or Region, on the same criteria as for equipment.

24. Some hospital staff, particularly nursing staff, either live close to hospitals in central urban areas or have homes too far distant for them to be easily recalled. Arrangements should therefore be made for such staff to be dispersed to evacuated convalescent homes, nursing homes or other accommodation on the fringe of the urban area. Suitable accommodation should be earmarked and transport planned.

25. Staff may be recalled, during a period of conventional war, to augment the emergency service of their hospital, but the numbers should be kept to the minimum required to deal with the casualties and no general recall should be ordered. After a nuclear attack, radioactive fall-out, either in the area or drifting towards it, might be at lethal or near lethal levels. It would be essential that staff, vital to the long term recovery of the country, should not be wasted by allowing them to enter areas of high radioactivity and no staff should leave shelter until authorised to do so by the District Controller (see paragraph 36). Hospitals from which the staff are originally dispersed might have been destroyed or isolated, or might not be best placed to handle the majority of casualties. When release from cover had been authorised, dispersed staff should report immediately to the nearest district general hospital. If this were no longer possible, staff should report to their nearest Casualty Collecting Centre (see paragraph 60). As the situation became clear, staff might be redeployed to augment other hospitals or casualty collecting centres.

Hospitals not vested in the Secretary of State

26. When empowered by an Order under Defence Regulations, the

Secretary of State may authorise AHAs to assume full control over all private hospitals, nursing homes and convalescent homes in the Area. At the discretion of the AHA, these establishments would be treated, for the purposes of the dispersal of patients, staff and supplies, in the same way as Health Service establishments.

General medical practitioners

27. Before an attack, the return of hospital patients to their homes would increase the work of the general practitioners and, after an attack, they would be fully engaged in caring for casualties and the sick in the community. General practitioners should not normally be employed in hospitals after the start of the dispersal of patients, nor should health authorities rely, other than in very exceptional circumstances, on general practitioners to augment the staff of hospitals after an attack. Exceptions, both before and after an attack would be those general practitioners who work in hospitals, particularly Community Hospitals, which are entirely dependent upon their services. General practitioners and their staff, if any, should be assigned to a Casualty Collecting Centre in their neighbourhood (paragraph 60), to which they should report immediately movement is allowed after an attack.

Dental practitioners

28. Health authorities should consider how best to employ the medical skills of dental practitioners. While some might be assigned to hospitals, following an attack, the majority might best be employed to assist in the care and sorting of casualties at a Casualty Collecting Centre. After an attack, as soon as radiological conditions allowed, dental practitioners should, unless otherwise arranged, report to the Casualty Collecting Centre in their neighbourhood.

Domiciliary services

29. The domiciliary services would continue to function normally until an attack. The return of hospital patients and the withdrawal of out-patient facilities would increase the work of the domiciliary services and health authorities should consider the augmentation of these services from dispersed hospital staff, particularly midwives. Each member of the domiciliary services should be assigned to a Domiciliary Team which should report, as soon as movement was allowed, to the doctor in charge of the Casualty Collecting Centre for the neighbourhood.

Individual volunteers

30. It may be expected that, during a period of crisis, many individuals with knowledge of first aid would offer their services. Volunteers should normally be directed to a Voluntary Aid Society which could assign them to a proposed First Aid Post (see paragraph 59) near their homes. In addition, a national appeal would be made to all those with medical or nursing qualifications, which they were not exercising, to report to their nearest Casualty Collecting Centre (see paragraph 60) as soon after an attack as movement was allowed.

Medical supplies

31. Action would be taken by the Department, prior to an attack, to arrange the distribution to health authorities of any centrally held medical supplies. After an attack, all supplies held by pharmacies, chemists, other retailers and wholesalers, would be requisitioned for the health services and made available to the public only in the course of medical treatment through general practitioners and Domiciliary Teams. Further supplies might not be available for many months and the most stringent economy of existing supplies would be essential. Further guidance on the distribution of supplies, including the medical stock pile will be given in due course.

Community Health Councils

32. During the transition to war of the health service, involving the discharge of patients and the dispersal of hospital staff, the activities of CHCs may be suspended by direction of the Secretary of State and would be suspended in the event of a nuclear attack. The staff of CHCs would be redeployed at the discretion of the Health Authority.

PART II — ORGANISATION FOR WAR

The machinery of government

33. England is divided into 9 Home Defence Regions, each containing one or more Sub-Regions (ES1/1973) and Commissioners would be appointed in war to exercise the functions of government (ES7/1973). Staff would be appointed from the Department, to Regional and Sub-Regional headquarters (see also paragraph 46).

34. Below Sub-Region, the processes of government in war would be

carried out at County and District level. (In London groups of London Boroughs would equate with County level). Each County and District has appointed a Controller (designate) (normally the Chief Executive) who would be empowered in war to exercise the full functions of government in his area. A chain of government could thus be established from the Region (when operational) through Sub-Region and County to District, supported by a network of communications.

35. The County or London Group Controller would determine priorities, plan for the most effective use of surviving resources in the County and co-ordinate the activities of essential services. The decisions of the County Controller would directly affect the provision and operation of health services and vice versa, and very close liaison between the County Controller and the appropriate level in the Health Service would be essential.

36. The District or London Borough Controller would have similar powers and responsibilities within his District and would be answerable to the County Controller, and, through him, to the Commissioner at Sub-Region and later, at Region. A very close liaison between the District Controller and the Health Service would also be essential.

Health Service organisation

37. The peace-time organisation of the Health Service does not lend itself to the rapid taking of decisions of the sort required in a war situation. It will be necessary therefore to provide for a control structure from the Commissioner through Health Service Regions, Areas and Districts to Sectors and Units, and for effective liaison with the appropriate County or District Controller at each level. Health Authorities, including Boards of Governors should therefore appoint a Health Director (Designate) to assume in war responsibility for all the Authority's functions; the responsibility for the preparation of the Authority's war plans rests with the authority itself who will delegate to their officers as appropriate.

Regional Health Director (RHD)

38. RHAs should now appoint their Regional Medical Officer as Regional Health Director (designate) and arrange to delegate to him when so directed by the Secretary of State, or in the event of enemy action destroying communications with the Department, full responsibility for the framing and execution of policy.

39. In peace-time the RHA would be responsible for the co-ordination of AHA plans and the preparation of the Region's plans for war, in accordance with the Department's directives. In consultation with the Controller (designate) of any Metropolitan County within the Region, the Authority should plan for liaison officers to the County's war time Control. In war, the Director would assume full responsibility for all Health Service functions in his Region, taking such action as he considered appropriate through other members of the Regional team of Officers, who would be answerable to him. He would be responsible for assessing the resources of the Health Service available to the Region; determining priorities in the allocation or re-allocation of resources; he would act in consultation and co-ordination with the appropriate Sub-Regions and County headquarters and would liaise as necessary with neighbouring RHDs. The Director would be directly answerable to the Commissioners at the Sub-Regions and later, the Regions, insofar as these included a part of the RHA. It is accepted that initially a RHD might have to be answerable for parts of his Region to more than one Commissioner, but adjustments to the Health Service Regional Boundaries would not be made until after an attack, when the extent of the destruction and the loss of communications might well dictate a realignment.

Area Health Directors (AHD)

40. AHAs should now appoint their Area Medical Officer as Area Health Director (designate) and arrange to delegate to him, when so directed or should communications be destroyed, full responsibility for the framing and execution of Area policy.

41. In peace-time the AHA would be responsible for the preparation and submission to the RHA, of Area plans for war and for taking preparatory measures in accordance with the advice of the RHA and Department's directives. The Authority, in consultation with Controllers (designate) of any Non-Metropolitan Counties and Metropolitan Districts should plan for liaison officers for their war-time control. In war, the Director would assume full responsibility for the health services in the Area, taking such action as he considered appropriate through other members of the Area Team of Officers who would be answerable to him. He would be responsible for assessing the Health Service resources available to the Area and determining a casualty policy. He would take action in consultation and co-ordination with the appropriate County or District Controller. He would maintain as far as he was able, communications with

the RHD and his DHDs and would liaise with neighbouring Area and District Health Directors. He would report and be answerable to the RHD, or in his absence, to the Commissioner at Sub-Region. He might delegate any of his functions to District Health Directors.

District Health Directors (DHD)

42. AHAs should appoint District Community Physicians as District Health Directors (designate). District Management Teams would draw up their war plans as directed by the AHA; this would in the case of non-metropolitan counties include the plans for liaison officers at the local authority's District war-time Control. In war, the 'District Health Director would carry out such functions as might be delegated to him by the AHD and would be responsible to the AHD for the execution of the Area casualty policy in the Health District. In the absence of the AHD he would assume full responsibility for the deployment of resources within his health District and, in consultation and co-ordination with the appropriate District Controllers, for the implementation of a casualty policy.

Sector and Unit Health Directors (SHD and UHD)

43. AHAs and Boards of Governors in consultation with the appropriate AHA should arrange for an officer in each Sector and Unit to prepare in peace, war emergency plans for the hospitals and establishments in his Sector or Unit and in war to assume full responsibility under the DHD or AHD, for those establishments. As arranged by the AHD or DHD he would establish liaison with the appropriate District Controller. In the absence of the AHD or DHD he would, in consultation and co-operation with the District Controller, take such action as seemed appropriate.

Special hospitals

44. When directed by the Secretary of State or in the event of an attack severing communications with the Department, special hospitals would come under the control of the AHD in whose area the hospital was situated. A Unit Health Director (designate) will be appointed for each hospital and be responsible in peace for any planning required by the AHA concerned, but should submit his plans to the Department for approval. In war, the Unit Health Director would be responsible to the AHD for the conduct of his

hospital. Patients should after an attack be discharged only on the authority of a Commissioner at Region or Sub-Region.

Community hospitals

45. Few community hospitals have, so far, been established and guidance about how they might be fitted into the health service organisation in war will have to wait until more knowledge has been gained about how they will operate in peace and the type of patients they will hold. Meanwhile, AHAs with such hospitals in their area should consider how they should be used following an attack. They might, for example, provide accommodation for a casualty collecting centre (see paragraph 60), be staffed as a casualty hospital or used as a hostel for patients, particularly the elderly, who could not otherwise be discharged.

Representation at Sub-Region

46. In addition to the officers appointed from the Department (paragraph 33) each RHA will appoint an administrator and a medical officer to the appropriate Sub-Regional Headquarters. The majority of RHAs cover parts of the area of more than one Sub-Region and further guidance will be given about the appointments to be made.

Liaison with County and District Controllers

47. The importance of establishing liaison between health authorities and County and District Controllers (designate) has been stressed. Difficulties arise however, because the boundaries of RHAs and Health Districts do not necessarily match Home Defence Regions or local authority boundaries respectively and AHA boundaries may be co-terminous with two different types of local authority i.e. County or Metropolitan District. A further difficulty arises in London, where London Boroughs are grouped under five Controllers (ES7/73) and AHAs may cover the area of more than one local authority not all of which will necessarily be in the same group. Any attempt to alter Health Authority boundaries to provide for easier liaison, would create administrative difficulties during a period of crisis and boundaries might in any case need adjustment following an

attack. Health authorities must accept that they would have to liaise with several local authorities of different types and responsibility lies with Health Authorities to plan for effective liaison in war with the County and District Controllers in their area.

48. Non-Metropolitan Counties. AHAs are co-terminous with the areas of non-Metropolitan Counties and the AHA should establish liaison with the County Controller (designate). AHAs should also arrange, if necessary through District Management Teams, for liaison with District Controllers.

49. Metropolitan Counties. AHAs are co-terminous with Metropolitan Districts and should establish liaison with the District Controller (designate). RHAs should arrange for liaison with the Controllers (designate) of the Metropolitan Counties.

50. London. AHAs should liaise with the London Boroughs they cover and RHAs should liaise with the London Groups. The three Northern London Groups consist of the London Boroughs covered by North East and North West Thames RHAs and the two Southern London Groups by South East and South West Thames RHAs. Each RHA should establish liaison with the London Group covering the majority of their area, but North East Thames RHA should liaise with both North West and North London Groups. This liaison must not be allowed to affect the line of control between RHA and its own AHAs.

Liaison officers

51. AHAs should consult with the appropriate County or District Controllers (designate) about the number of liaison officers required and their location before an attack; which will depend on the situation of their respective headquarters; the space available at the local authority headquarters and other local factors. The aim should be to establish effective liaison in war between the Director and the Controller, which would provide the former with information about the post attack situation in his areas and advice on the resources and intentions of the Controller, and provide the latter with information about the resources and capabilities of the Health Service to deal with casualties and advice on the health and care of the community. Liaison officers should therefore be able to advise on medical, nursing and administrative matters and, ideally, one officer from each of these branches of the Health Service should be appointed, although, in practice, this might not be feasible.

Joint Consultative Committees

52. JCCs provide a valuable link between health and local authorities in peacetime and might be able to foster co-operation and encourage progress in joint planning. They would have no role once hostilities began and they would remain in abeyance for several months at least, until the longer-term decisions on the future of the health service and local government were taken.

Medical advice for local authority functions

53. NHS Medical Officers appointed by local authorities as 'proper officers' for their environmental health functions, should remain with their local authority as medical advisers to the Controllers. These officers would be very fully employed and should not, in addition, be appointed by health authorities as their liaison officers with the local authorities. Where a Doctor has been appointed as 'proper officer' by more than one local authority, or the DCP as District Health Director (designate) is himself a 'proper officer' the AHA and the local authority should jointly agree the nomination of additional doctors so that, in war, each District Councillor would have his own medical adviser on public and environmental health.

PART III—CASUALTY POLICY

General

54. This Part suggests how the preparatory measures and the organisation for war of the Health Service, set out in the preceding Parts, might be applied to a situation following an attack. The detailed procedures by which resources might best be applied to achieve the aims of the Health Service in war, however, require to be evolved through consultations between Health Directors and County and District Controllers; seminars and exercises with Health Authorities and at the Home Defence College and discussions between the departments and services concerned. The proposals in this Part are designed to provide a frame-work on which health authorities can build their plans. Further guidance will be given as procedures are developed.

55. As explained in paragraphs 5 to 7 above; radiological conditions may be expected to prevent any organised life saving operation for

days or weeks following an attack. Trained health service staff would be vital to the future and should not be wasted by allowing them to enter areas of high contamination where casualties would, in any case, have small chance of long term recovery. County and District Controllers would receive information about radio-active intensities in their area, forecasts about the decay rate and predictions of further fall-out, carried by wind, from other areas of destruction. The Health Director should liaise with the Controller to find out when and for how long, measures to avoid further loss of life could be taken in the open. In areas of great destruction, with a consequent loss of communications, the Health Director concerned might, initially, be the Sector, or even Unit, Director.

56. No Director would be able to rely on receiving or giving assistance to neighbouring Authorities and, in the first instance, would have to concentrate on making the best arrangements possible with the resources available to him. As Directors at successive levels were able to review the situation over wider areas, arrangements could be made for the transfer of casualties to make the best use of all available resources and to relieve the areas hardest hit.

57. When movement became possible, emphasis would have to be placed on self help, with minor injuries being treated by relatives or friends, to avoid overburdening the health services with cases of superficial injury. More serious casualties would be treated as First Aid Posts (FAPs), established by the Voluntary Aid Societies. Casualties requiring further treatment would be sent to nearby Casualty Collecting Centres (CCCs) run by general medical practitioners with the assistance of Domiciliary Teams (see para 30) and volunteers. CCCs would treat and sort casualties for priority admission to hospital, return to the community or temporary retention. The resources available to the health services however would dictate that the majority of casualties would have to be cared for by relatives, friends or volunteers, in their own homes or local authority rest centres, with assistance from general practitioners and members of the Domiciliary Teams based on the CCCs.

The collection of casualties

58. The Regional or Area Health Director concerned would be responsible for the deployment of ambulances but, in his absence, the highest Director able to exercise control would take this responsibility. Additional vehicles might be obtained by requisition, in

conjunction with the County or District Controller. In high casualty areas however, no arrangements for the deployment of ambulances could deal adequately with the numbers involved. The immediate collection and transport of casualties would be a matter for the public themselves and it may be expected that, as soon as movement became possible, there would be a substantial flow of casualties into First Aid Posts. As ambulances became available they could be concentrated on clearing the more distant and difficult areas, but Directors would need to attach ambulances to CCCs to collect casualties from FAPs and to deliver priority cases to hospitals.

First Aid Posts

59. AHAs should plan with the Voluntary Aid Societies in their area for the establishment and manning of FAPs as soon after an attack as possible. These Posts should be set up to provide cover for the whole area and should be located next to local authority rest centres; in Health Service property (such as health centres and clinics and vacated convalescent and nursing homes) and in property earmarked in peace with the Controllers (designate) for immediate requisition in war. The purpose of FAPs would be to give immediate treatment and to sort casualties into those who could be returned home or to a rest centre, and those requiring further treatment at a CCC.

Casualty Collecting Centres

60. The number of casualties may be expected greatly to exceed surviving hospital resources and Directors would have to impose strict admission priorities. Casualty Collecting Centres would therefore be established, between the FAPs and the hospitals to treat, sort and hold casualties until they could be accepted by a hospital. CCCs should be set up in each neighbourhood, in premises previously earmarked, near to but separate from FAPs and local authority rest centres. Each CCC should be staffed by 4 to 6 general medical practitioners, normally practising in the area, and one of the GPs should be appointed doctor in charge. The GPs should be assisted by the local Domiciliary Team (see paragraph 30), and volunteers. As soon as any FAP could be closed, the staff should be redeployed to augment a CCC. Medical supplies would be obtained from requisitioned stocks. Ambulance vehicles should be attached to CCCs to collect casualties from FAPs (if the distance required it) and to convey priority cases to hospitals. CCCs would, initially,

have no administrative organisation and Directors would have to arrange with District Controllers for the provision of food, and, if necessary, of water; medical supplies from requisitioned stocks; kitchen and unskilled staff and the removal and burial of the dead.

61. CCCs would undertake emergency treatment, including minor surgical procedures. A main function however would be to sort casualties into those who could be returned home or to a rest centre, after treatment; those who should have priority for admission to hospital, and non-priority and radiation only cases who, for the time being, would have to be retained. Treatment and care would have to be simple and improvised. Casualties retained at a CCC would have to provide as much basic nursing care for each other as their injuries allowed.

Hospitals

62. Despite any damage and the disruption of public utilities and service, the surviving hospitals might be expected to offer the best facilities for surgical procedures. The Director would have to enforce strict priorities for the admission of casualties to prevent hospitals being overwhelmed. In general, hospitals should, initially, accept only those casualties who, after limited surgical procedures, would be likely to be alive after seven days, with a fair chance of eventual recovery. The more complete the recovery that could be expected, the higher the priority for admission. People suffering from radiation sickness only, should not be admitted. There is no specific treatment for radiation injury, although spontaneous recovery may be assisted by good nursing, and all radiation cases should be nursed in the community. Hospitals would call forward priority cases from CCCs as space for their treatment became available. Casualties would be returned to the community as soon as their clinical condition allowed.

Domiciliary services

63. The majority of casualties would have to be cared for in their own homes or in a local authority rest centre, by relatives, friends or volunteers. GPs and members of the Domiciliary Team at a CCC would visit casualties, at the discretion of the doctor in charge, to assist in their care. Members of Domiciliary Teams could not themselves however undertake the continuing care of casualties in the community. Their purpose would be to advise and assist those caring for the casualties; to carry out certain nursing procedures;

to provide drugs and dressings; to advise the Director, through the doctor in charge of the CCC, of cases which should have priority for admission to hospital and of the general casualty situation in the community.

Planning

64. The plan of action set out in this circular is as simple as a realistic approach to the problems of placing the health service on a war footing allows and should be capable of being implemented, if necessary, within a relatively short period of time. The more pre-planning that can be done the more complete and effective would be the transition to war of the Health Authorities, although it is appreciated that Health Authorities may not, at present, be in a position to undertake much detailed planning. The following paragraphs outline the main action that should be taken as time and resources permit. Any plans must be co-ordinated with those of the local authorities and should therefore be prepared in consultation with the appropriate Controller (designate).

Designation of Health Directors

65. Regional and Area Health Authorities should designate their Directors; the latter should also designate Directors for health districts and, as necessary, arrange for designation of Directors for Sectors and Units. Boards of Governors should, similarly, designate Directors for their own hospitals.

Regional plans

66. RHAs should arrange for the preparation and subsequent co-ordination of plans for their Region, for:
    a. discharging patients,
    b. dispersing medical supplies and equipment, blood supplies, ambulances and staff,
    c. forming Domiciliary Teams,
    d. taking control of private establishments,
    e. liaising with local authorities,
    f. appointing medical advisers to local authority Controllers,
and
    g. dealing with casualties.

Area plans

67. AHA's should prepare their contribution to the Regional plan as may be required by the RHA and, in particular, should arrange with:

a. The Voluntary Aid Societies, for the setting up of FAPs and the staffing of CCCs,

b. the Family Practitioner Committee for the assignment of GPs to CCCs

and

c. local authority Controllers (designate), for liaison and for the earmarking for requisition, of medical supplies, vehicles and accommodation, not in the ownership or occupation of the NHS and its servants.

Training

68. The Home Defence College offers places, through the Department, on courses and seminars. Health Authorities should accept as many places as possible to give their staff a background to home defence policy which will enable them to contribute to discussions on the development of casualty policies. As plans are completed they should be made known to all staff in senior and middle level posts.

References

1. Committee for the Compilation of Materials on Damage Caused by the Atomic Bombings in Hiroshima and Nagasaki. *Hiroshima and Nagasaki: The Physical, Medical and Social Effects of the Atomic Bombings*. Trans. Ishikawa, E. and Swain, D. L., London, Hutchinson, 1981.

2. Glasstone, S. and Dolan, P. J. (eds). *The Effects of Nuclear Weapons*. United States Department of Defence and United States Department of Energy. 3rd edn 1977. Published in UK by Castle House, Tunbridge Wells, 1980.

3. Rotblat, J. *Nuclear Radiation in Warfare*. London, Taylor and Francis, 1981.

4. Department of Political and Security Council Affairs United Nations Centre for Disarmament: Report of the Secretary General. *Comprehensive Study on Nuclear Weapons*. New York, United Nations, 1981.

5. United Nations, Report of the Secretary General. *Nuclear Weapons*. London, Frances Pinter, 1981.

6. Stockholm International Peace Research Institute, Yearbook 1974. *World Armaments and Disarmament*. London, Taylor and Francis, 1974.

7. Goodwin, P. *Nuclear War: The Facts on Our Survival*. London, Ash and Grant, 1981.

8. International Institute for Strategic Studies. *The Military Balance 1980-81*. London, IISS, 1980.

9. Clarke, M. *The Nuclear Destruction of Britain*. London, Croom Helm, 1982.

10. Stockholm International Peace Research Institute, Yearbook 1980. *World Armaments and Disarmament*. London, Taylor and Francis, 1980.

11. International Institute for Strategic Studies. *The Military Balance 1979-80*. London, IISS, 1980.

12. Stockholm International Peace Research Institute, Yearbook, 1982. *World Armaments and Disarmament*. London, Taylor and Francis, 1982.

13. International Institute for Strategic Studies. *The Military Balance 1982-83*. London, IISS, 1982.

14. Peterson, J. (ed.). *AMBIO, A Journal of the Human Environment*. Royal Swedish Academy of Sciences/Pergamon Press, 1982, **XI**, Number 2-3.

15. Openshaw, S. and Steadman, P. 'On the geography of a worst case nuclear attack on the population of Britain'. *Political Geography Quarterly*, July 1982, **3**, 263-278.

16. Clayton, J. K. S. *Training Manual for Scientific Advisors*, Scottish Home and Health Department. Edinburgh, HMSO, 1978.

17. Home Office and Central Office of Information, *Domestic Nuclear Shelters: Technical Guidance*. London, HMSO, 1981.

18. Butler, S. F. J. 'Scientific advice in Home Defence' in Barnaby, C. F. and Thomas, G. P. (eds), *The Nuclear Arms Race: Control or Catastrophe*. London, Frances Pinter, 1982.

19. Rogers, P. 'Possible Nuclear Attack Scenarios on Britain' in Dando, M. R. and Newman, B. R. (eds) *Nuclear Deterrence: Implications and Policy Options for the 1980s*, pp.137-145. Tunbridge Wells, Castle House, 1982.

20. Openshaw, S. and Steadman, P. 'On the geography of the bomb', paper presented to conference of the Institute of British Geographers, Edinburgh, 5-8 January 1983.

21. Zuckerman, S. *Nuclear Illusion and Reality*. London, Collins, 1982.

22. Sokolovskii, V. D. (ed.) *Military Strategy*. 3rd edn Moscow, Military Publishing House, 1968.

23. Andrews, G. A. 'Medical Management of Accidental Total Body Irradiation' in Hubner, K. F. and Fry, J. A. (eds) *The Medical Basis for Radiation Accident Preparedness*. Elsevier, North Holland, 1980.

24. Miller, R. W. and Blot, W. J. 'Small head size after in utero exposure to atomic radiation'. *Lancet* 1972, **2**, p.784.

25. Haynes, A. P. 'Possible consequences of a nuclear attack on London' in Chivian, E., Chivian, S., Lifton, R. J. and Mack, J. E. (eds) *Last Aid*. San Francisco, W. H. Freeman and Co., 1983.

26. Orth, G. L. 'Disaster and Disposal of the Dead' *Military Medicine* 1959, **124**, pp.505-510.

27. Hachiya, M. *Hiroshima Diary: The Journal of a Japanese Physician, August 6-September 30, 1945*. Tokyo, Asahi Shimbursha, 1955.

28. Lifton, R. J. and Olsen, E. 'Human meaning of total disaster. The Buffalo Creek Experience'. *Psychiatry* 1976, **39**, pp.1-18.

29. Office of Technology Assessment, Congress of the United States. *The Effects of Nuclear War*. London, Croom Helm, 1980.

30. Qasrawi, A., Wellhoefer, F. and Steward, F. *Ground Zero: The Short-term Effects of a Nuclear Attack on the West Midlands*. Scientists against Nuclear Arms, 1982.

31. Greene, O., Rubin, B., Turok, N., Webber, P., Wilkinson, G. *London After the Bomb*. Oxford, Oxford University Press, 1982.

32. Home Office and Central Office of Information. *Protect and Survive*. London, HMSO, 1980.

33. Openshaw, S. and Steadman, P. 'Predicting the consequences of a nuclear attack on Britain: Models, results and public policy implications', *Environment and Planning C*, in press.

34. Bentley, P. R. *Blast overpressure and fall-out radiation dose models for casualty assessment and other purposes*. Home Office Scientific Research and Development Branch, 1981.

35. Home Office and Scottish Home and Health Department. *Nuclear Weapons*. 3rd edn London, HMSO, 1974.
36. British Mission to Japan. *The Effects of the Atomic Bombs at Hiroshima and Nagasaki*. London, HMSO, 1946.
37. Butterfield, *et al*. 'Flash burns from atomic weapons'. *Surgery, Gynaecology and Obstetrics* 1956, **103**, 6, pp.655-665.
38. British Institute of Radiology. *Report of the BIR Working Party on the Radiological Effects of Nuclear War* 1982.
39. Parker, G. 'Cyclone Tracy and the Darwin Evacuees, on the Restoration of Species'. *British Journal of Psychiatry* 1977, **130**, pp.548-555.
40. Jackson, A. A. 'Feeding the United Kingdom After a Nuclear Attack: a preliminary review'. Thesis, unpublished, 1979.
41. US Environmental Protection Agency. *Air Quality Criteria for Ozone and other Photochemical Oxidants*. EPA—600/8-78-004. Washington DC, 1978.

Bibliography

Akizuki, Tatsuichiro. *Nagasaki 1945*, trans. Keiichi Nagata, Quartet, London 1981.

Alley, E. E. 'Emergency planning in the nuclear age", *Practitioner* 1981, **225**, pp.711-720.

Ambio (Journal of the Human Environment). Royal Swedish Academy of Sciences. Pergamon Press. **XI**, Number 2-3, 1982.

Barnaby, Frank. *Prospects for Peace*. Pergamon, Oxford 1980.

Barnaby, C. F. and Thomas, G. P. (eds). *The Nuclear Arms Race: Control or Catastrophe*. Paper presented at meeting of British Association for the Advancement of Science, York, September 1981. Frances Pinter, London 1982.

Bentley, P. R. 'Blast overpressure and fallout radiation dose models for casualty assessment and other purposes'. Home Office Scientific Research & Development Branch Report, 1981.

British Journal of Radiology March 1983. *Report of British Institute of Radiology*.

Broad, W. J. (three articles on EMP). 'Nuclear Pulse (I)', 'Nuclear Pulse (II): Ensuring Delivery of the Doomsday Signal', 'Nuclear Pulse (III): Playing a Wild Card'. *Science* 1981, **212**, pp.1116-20: 1248-51.

Burton, J. 'Dear Survivors . . .' Frances Pinter, London 1982.

Butler, S. F. J. 'Scientific advice in Home Defence', in Barnaby, C. F. and Thomas, G. P. (eds), *The Nuclear Arms Race: Control or Catastrophe* pp.135-163. London, Frances Pinter, 1982.

Butterfield *et al.* 'Flash burns from atomic weapons', *Surgery, Gynaecology and Obstetrics* 1956, **103**, 6, pp.655-665.

Campbell, Duncan. 'World War III: an exclusive preview', *New Statesman*, 3rd October, 1980.

Campbell, Duncan. 'Scotland's nuclear targets', *New Statesman*, 6th March, 1981.

Clarke, Magnus. *The Nuclear Destruction of Britain*. Croom Helm, London 1982.

Committee for the Compilation of Materials on Damage Caused by the Atomic Bombings in Hiroshima and Nagasaki. *Hiroshima and Nagasaki: The Physical, Medical and Social Effects of the Atomic Bombings*, trans. Eisei Ishikawa and D. L. Swain. Hutchinson, London 1981.

Department of Health and Social Security, Home Defence Circular HDC (77)1, 'The Preparation and Organisation of the Health Service for War', January 1977.

Drell, S. D. and von Hippel, Frank. 'Limited Nuclear War', *Scientific American* 1976, **235**, No. 5, pp.27-37.

Eastwood, Martin. 'The Medicine of Nuclear Warfare: A Clinical Dead-end', *The Lancet*, June 6, 1981, pp.1252-1253.

Electronics and Power. 'EMP—the forgotten threat?' July/August 1981.

Fetter, S. A. and Tsipis, Kosta. 'Catastrophic Releases of Radioactivity' *Scientific American* 1981, **244**, No. 4, pp.33-39.

Forsborg, R. 'Call to Halt the Nuclear Arms Race' 1980.

Gaskell, R. 'Nuclear Weapons: the way ahead'. The Menard Press 1981.

Geiger, J. H. 'Addressing Apocalypse Now: The effects of nuclear warfare as a public health concern', *American Journal of Public Health* 1980, **70**, pp.958-981.

Glasstone, Samuel and Dolan, Phillip, J. (eds). *The Effects of Nuclear Weapons*, United States Department of Defence and United States Department of Energy: 3rd edn, 1977. Published in England by Castle House, Tunbridge Wells, 1980.

Goodwin, Peter. *Nuclear War: The Facts on our Survival*. Ash and Grant, London 1981.

Hachiya, Michihiko. *Hiroshima Diary*. Asahi Shimbunsha, Tokyo 1955.

Hedge, A. 'Surviving a Nuclear War', *Proceedings of the Medical Association for the Prevention of War*, 1981, **3, 5**, pp.185-200.

Hersey, John. *Hiroshima*. Knopf, New York 1946. Penguin, Harmondsworth 1966.

Hiatt, H. H. 'Preventing the last epidemic', *Journal of the American Medical Association*, 1980, **244**, pp.2314-5.

Hiroshima and Nagasaki: A Pictorial Record of the Atomic Destruction. Hiroshima-Nagasaki Publishing Committee, Tokyo 1978.

Home Office Circular No. ES 7/1973. 'Machinery of Government in War: Planning Assumptions and General Guidance'.

Home Office and Scottish Home and Health Department. *Nuclear Weapons*. HMSO, London 3rd edn 1974.

Home Office 'Emergency Services' Division Circulars 1975: ES1/1975 'Nuclear Weapons', ES2/1975 'Information Services in War', ES3/1975 'Police Manual of Home Defence', ES4/1975 'Construction Work and Building Materials in War', ES5/1975 'Communications in War', ES6/1975 'Post Office Telephone Preference System', ES7/1975 'Major Accidents and Natural Disasters'.

Home Office and Central Office of Information. *Protect and Survive*. HMSO, London 1980.

Home Office and Central Office of Information. *Domestic Nuclear Shelters: Technical Guidance*. HMSO, London 1981.

Hubner, K. F. and Fry, S. A. (eds). *The Medical Basis for Radiation Accident Preparedness*. Elsevier, North Holland, 1980.

Ikle, Fred C. *The Social Impact of Bomb Destruction*. University of Oklahoma, Norman, Oklahoma 1958.

Ickle, Fred C. *Every War Must End* (Under Secretary of Defence for Policy). Proceedings of Conference on Understanding Nuclear War. Imperial College, London 1980.

International Institute for Strategic Studies. *The Military Balance 1980-1981*. IISS, London 1980.

Irving, David. *The Destruction of Dresden*. Kimber, London 1963.

Ishimaru, T. *et al.* 'Dose-response relationship of neutrons and gamma-rays to leukaemia among atomic bomb survivors in Hiroshima and Nagasaki by type of leukaemia 1950-1971', *Radiation Research* 1979, **77**, pp.377-394.

Japanese Broadcasting Corporation (NHK). *Unforgettable Fire: Pictures Drawn by Atomic Bomb Survivors*. Wildwood House, London 1981.

Jungk, Robert. *Brighter than a Thousand Suns*. Penguin, Harmondsworth 1964.

Kaplan, Fred M. *Dubious Specter: A Skeptical Look at the Soviet Nuclear Threat*. Institute for Policy Studies, Washington DC, 1977.

Katz, Arthur M. *Life After Nuclear War: The Economic and Social Impacts of Nuclear Attacks on the United States*. Ballinger, Cambridge Mass. 1982.

Kearny, C. H. *Nuclear War Survival Skills*. Oak Ridge National Laboratory, US Department of Commerce Technical Information Service 1979.

Laurie, P. *Beneath the City Streets*. Panther, London 1979.

Lewis, K. N. 'The prompt and delayed effects of nuclear war', *Scientific American* 1979, **241**, pp.27-39.

Liebow, A. *et al.* 'Pathology of the atomic bomb casualties', *American Journal of Pathology* 1949, **25**, pp.853-860.

Lifton, Robert J. *Death in Life—Survivors of Hiroshima*. Random House, New York 1967.

Lindop, Patricia J. 'Medical Consequences of Radioactive Fallout', paper presented to First Congress of International Physicians for the Prevention of Nuclear War, Airlie House, March 1981.

Lindop, Patricia J. 'Radiation Aspects of a Nuclear War in Europe', paper presented at Conference on Nuclear War in Europe, Groningen, The Netherlands, April 1981.

Lown, Bernard, Chivian, Eric, Muller, James and Abrams, Herbert. 'Sounding board: The nuclear arms race and the physician', *New England Journal of Medicine* March 19, 1981, pp.726-729.

Mack, J. E. 'Psychological Effects of the Nuclear Arms Race', *Bulletin of the Atomic Scientists*, April 1981.

Mark, J. Carson. 'Global Consequences of Nuclear Weaponry', *Annual Review of Nuclear Science* 1976, **26**, pp.51-87.

Medical Campaign against Nuclear Weapons, and Medical Association for the Prevention of War. *The Medical Consequences of Nuclear Weapons*. Cambridge 1981.

Morland, Howard. 'The H-bomb secret: To know how is to ask why', *The Progressive* November 1979, pp.14-23.

National Academy of Sciences. *Long-Term Worldwide Effects of Multiple Nuclear-Weapons Detonations*. NAS, Washington DC, 1975.

Neild, Robert. *How to make up your mind about the Bomb*. Deutsch, London 1981.

Britain and the Bomb. New Statesman papers on destruction and disarmament. New Statesman Report 3, London, 1981.

Office of Technology Assessment, Congress of the United States. *The Effects of Nuclear War*. Croom Helm, London 1980.

Openshaw, S. and Steadman, P. 'On the geography of a worst case nuclear attack on the population of Britain', *Political Geography Quarterly* July 1982, **3**.

Oughterson, A. W. and Warren, S. *Medical Effects of the Atomic Bomb in Japan*. McGraw-Hill, New York 1956.

Owen-Smith, M. S. 'Explosion blast injury', *Journal of the Royal Army Medical Corps*, 1979, **125**, pp.4-16.

Special study section of Physicians for Social Responsibility: 'The medical consequences of thermonuclear war', *New England Journal of Medicine* 1962, **266**, pp.1126-1155.

Ritchie, R. H. and Hurst, G. S. 'Penetration of weapons radiation — Application to the Hiroshima-Nagasaki studies', *Health Physics* 1959, **1**, 390.

Rotblat, J. 'Risks for radiation workers', *Bulletin of the Atomic Scientists* 1978, **34**, pp.41-46.

Rotblat, J., for Stockholm International Peace Research Institute. *Nuclear Radiation in Warfare*. Taylor and Francis, London 1981.

Proceedings of Conference on Medical Consequences of Nuclear Disaster, Royal Society of Medicine 1980.

Schell, Jonathan. *The Fate of the Earth*. Pan, London 1982.

Smith, Jane and Smith, Tony. 'Medicine and the Bomb.' Four articles: 'Nuclear War: the medical facts'; 'Radiation injury and effects of early fallout'; 'Long-term effects of radiation'; 'Attitudes towards civil defence and the psychological effects of nuclear war'. *British Medical Journal* 19 Sept 1981, **283**, pp.771-774; 26 Sept 1981, **283**, pp.844-846; 3 Oct 1981, **283**, pp.907-908; 10 Oct 1981, **283**, pp.963-965.

Steadman, Philip. 'The Bomb: Worse than Government Admits', *New Scientist* 1981, **90**, pp.769-771.

Stockholm International Peace Research Institute, Yearbook 1980, *World Armaments and Disarmament*. Taylor and Francis, London 1980.

Swiss Federal Department of Justice and Police Office of Civil Defense. *Technical Directives for the Construction of Private Air Raid Shelters* and *The 1971 Conception of the Swiss Civil Defense*. English Language editions republished by Oak Ridge National Laboratory, Tennessee ORNL-TR-2707.

United Nations. *Nuclear Weapons*. Report of the Secretary-General.

US Arms Control and Disarmament Agency. *An Analysis of Civil Defense in Nuclear War*. ACDA, Washington DC, 1978.

United States Strategic Bombing Survey. *The Effects of Atomic Bombs on Hiroshima and Nagasaki.* Pacific War Reports No. 3, US Government Printing Office, Washington DC, 1946.

Westing, Arthur H. 'Neutron Bombs and the Environment', *Ambio* 1978, **7**, No. 3, pp.93-97.

Zuckerman, Solly. *Nuclear Illusion and Reality.* Collins, London 1982.

Index

A-bombs 2
Abdominal injuries 40
Absorbed dose xiii
Accident and Emergency Departments (*see* Casualty Departments)
Accidental irradiation 33
Accidents 33
  Nuclear Power Industry 110
  schemes for civilians 39
Accuracy/Circular Error Probability (CEP) 10
Acute exposure 81
Aggression/Anger 37
Agriculture 94, 99, 123
Air burst 8, 15, 31, 41, 52, 58, 60, 63
Air-raids 38
All clear signal 77
Alpha radiation xiii
Ambulance Services 12, 38, 39
Anaesthetics 42
Analgesics 42
Anorexia 33
Anti-emetics 42
Antibiotics 40, 42
Anxiety, 37, 76
Apathy 37
Arms Control and Disarmament Research Unit of the Foreign and Commonwealth Office 28
Arsenals (*see* Nuclear arsenals)
Arthritis 43
Atmosphere 12, 69, 98, 123
Atmospheric tests 9
Attack (patterns of) 15, 56, 74
'Average' nuclear attack 15-30, 92, 107

Ballistic missiles (ICBM) (IRMB) 10, 78
Barnaby 25, 29, 51, 53
Basement 74, 75, 76
Bentley 89
Bereavement 36
Beta radiation xiii
Blast 4, 31, 32, 57, 61, 66, 70, 71, 78, 79, 121
Blast casualties 57, 61, 66, 90
Blood 41, 44
  count 42
  granulocyte count 34
  lymphocytes 33

lymphopoenia 33
  plasma 39, 44
  platelets 34, 42
  products/transfusion 124
  transfusion 43, 44, 115
  white cells 42
Board of Science and Education x, 125
Bone marrow 88
  damage 33, 38
  transplantation 33, 34, 42
Breakdown of medical facilities 41
Brief exposure 84
Britain (*see* United Kingdom)
British Institute of Radiology 82, 88
British Medical Association (BMA) ix
British Medical Journal (BMJ) 38
British Mission to Japan 67
Buffalo Creek flood 37
Bungalow 74, 75
Burns 4, 32, 35, 39, 41, 55, 69, 70, 79, 91, 122
Butler 48-63, 68, 70, 78, 90

Caesium 137, 96
Calorie intake 97
Cancer 33
Carcinogenesis 103
Casualty collecting centres 115
Casualty Departments/Accident and Emergency Departments 36, 39
Casualty estimation 61, 68, 70, 73
Casualty numbers 38-79
Causes of death 103
Cereal production 95, 123
Chain reaction 2
Chemical explosion 32, 66
Chemical pollution 98
Cholera 101, 102
Chromosome aberrations 104
Chronic bronchitis 43
Circular Error Probability (CEP) 10
City centres 56, 58
City targets 78
Civil defence (*see* Home defence)
Civilian disaster 129
Clayton 97
Clothing 116

Collapse (of buildings) 75
Communicable disease 40, 100, 123
Communications 14, 24, 39
Compton electrons 14
Computer Studies — Home Office 22, 60, 79, Figure 3.7
  Openshaw and Steadman 22, 52-58, 70-79
  model 24, 48, 52, 55, 56, 61, 72, 77, 79, Figure 3.7
Confusion 37
Conventional bombs 28
Corpses 39, 42
Counterforce 18, 55, 78, 91
County controller 106
Crater 9
Critical mass 2, 7
Crop damage 96
Crop harvest 99
Crop yield 98
Cross wind 72
Cruise missiles 10, 24, 25, 29
Crush injuries 4, 32
'Cyclone Tracy' 37

DHSS 112, 119
Damage rings 59-65, 79
Defence bases 106
Deficiency disease 123
Degradation Effect 79
Dehydration 101
Delays in treatment 39
'Demonstration attack' 117, 118
Deposition region 14
Depression 37
Deterrence 27, 28, 120
Detroit and Leningrad (DTA study) 57, 58, 70
Deuterium 7
Diabetes 43, 122
Diarrhoea 34, 36, 101
Diarrhoeal diseases 101
Dietary pattern 123
Diphtheria 102
Discrepancies 4, 20, 59-68, 121
District controller 106
Dolan (Glasstone and) 47-73
Domestic Nuclear Shelter: Technical Guidance (1981) 63
Dose equivalent xiii
Dose rate 34, 87
Dose/injury model 73
Drugs 43, 44, 123
  anaesthetics 42
  analgesics 42
  anti-emetics 42
  antibiotics 40, 42
  ferrotyne 44
  increased production 43
  lack of
  manufacture 43, 44, 124
  morphine 42
  penicillin 44

  phosphine 44
  quinines 44
  steroid 44
  stocks 43
  sulphonamides 44

'Earthquake' effect 9
Economic cost 121
Electro-magnetic pulse (EMP) 12
Energy 4, 5, 32
Energy supply 100
Enhanced Radiation Weapons (Neutron bombs) 17
Enteric diseases 104
Enteric infectious diseases 102
Erythema (see Radiation erythema)
Escalation 15, 26, 29, 118, 120
Evacuation 39, 56, 106, 121
Exercise ARC 63, 64, Figure 3.1
Explosive lenses.2
Explosive yield/Explosive power 45-66
Exposure — to heat and fire 39
  to radiation 33
  to wet and cold 39

Fall-out 9, 31-79
  area affected 41, 72
  contours 72
  size of particles 72
  standard methods of prediction 71
  water supply 92, 93
  window sills 76
Farm animals 96
'Fat man' 2
Ferrotyne 44
Fertility 35
Fertilizers 99
Fire alarm 70
Fireball 8, 32, 70
Fires 41, 71
  fighting 71
Firestorm 32, 71
First aid 39
First Aid Posts 114
Fission 1
Fluid replacement 92
Food-chains 96
  emergency supplies 39, 40, 76, 94, 122
  dumps 107
  palatability 123
  processing and distribution 94
  production 94
  stockpiles 94
  supplies 94, 99, 122
Forest fires 97
Fuel 100
Fuel/power 40, 92, 122
Fusion 6

Gamma rays 33, 74
Gastro-enteritis 36
Gastro-intestinal symptoms 34

Genetic effects 104
Germany 17, 24, 27
Glasstone and Dolan 47-73
Government 99, 106, 121
  devolution 106
  planning 112
Granulocyte count 34
Greer 109
Ground burst 8, 15, 33, 58-74
Ground zero 6, 32, 59, 62
Guidance systems 9, 10
'Gun' technique 3

H-bombs (see Thermonuclear)
Haemorrhage 92
Hair loss 35
Health 100
Health Service 40, 112
Heat/light 5, 6, 31, 39, 69, 121
Helium 7
Herbal remedies 45
Herbicides 99
Hiroshima 1, 34-124
Home Office 22, 48-79, 121, 122
Home defence ix, 43, 72, 92, 105, 121
Home defence regions 106
Hospital beds 36, 38, 39, 41, 42, 43, 113
House construction, UK 68, 71, 78
House construction, USA 68
Houses 74, 75, 78
  basements 74, 75, 76
  bungalow 74, 75
  collapse 74, 75
  detached 74, 75
  flats 74, 75
  semi-detached 74, 75
  terraced 74, 75
  upper storeys 74, 75
Hypothermia 102
Hypothyroidism 104
Hysteria 36

Immune defences 84, 100
Immunisation 40, 43, 100
Imponderables 21
Infant mortality 123
Infection 100
  secondary 34-43, 92
Initial radiation 6
Inuries 70
  abdominal 40
  burns (see Burns)
  crush 4, 32
  long term 103, 122
  orthopaedic 40
  psychological 35, 42, 108
  short term 34
  synergistic 45
  thoracic 40
Insects 96, 102
Intercontinental ballistic missiles (ICBM's) 17, 78

Intermediate range weapons 17, 22, 123
Iodine 96, 131
Ionising radiation — X-rays 31, 58, 74
Ionosphere 12

Japan (see also Hiroshima and Nagasaki) 3

Keloids 32

LD-50 33, 81, 96
'Launch on warning' 29
Leningrad (Detroit and Leningrad OTA Study) 57
Lethality 10, 18
Leukaemia 103
Limited attack 25, 26
Lindop 82, 88
'Little Boy' 1
Livestock 95
London After the Bomb Group 84, Table 3.5
Long term effects 103, 122
Lord Mountbatten 26, 28
Lower yield weapon 57, 91
Lown 109
Lymphocytes 33
Lymphopoenia 33

Mach wave 8
Malaria 102
Malignant conditions 43, 104
Malnutrition 100
Manila 42
Marrow, J. 63, 69
Marshall Islanders 35
Mean marrow dose 87
Measles 102
Median lethal dose (LD-50) 33, 81, 96
Medical conditions — arthritis 43
  cancer/malignant disease 43, 104
  chronic bronchitis 43
  diabetes 43, 122
  infection 43
  pregnancy 43
  renal disease 108
  strokes 43
Medical effects/injuries 25, 120-124
  abdominal 40
  burns (see Burns)
  crush injuries 4, 32
  long term 103
  orthopaedic 40
  psychiatric 38, 102
  psychological 35, 42, 108
  short term 34
  synergistic 45
  thoracic 40
Medical practitioners 40, 41, 124
Medical staff 40, 41, 42
Medical supplies 41, 123
Mental retardation 35
Microcephaly 35

Military targets 18, 78, 91
Milk 96
Minerals 97
Ministry of Defence 23, 27
Mitosis 34
Morphine 42
Multiple independently targetable re-entry vehicle (MIRV) 9

NATO 17, 23
Nagasaki 2, 34-124
National Health Service 38, 112, 113-119, 124
    wartime role 113
National Radiological Protection Board (NRPB) 83
Nausea 33, 36, 42
Neurovascular syndrome 34
Neutron 2, 34
    radiation 34
Northern Hemisphere 123
Nuclear arsenal ix, 15, 16, 57
Nuclear attack 15, 36, 39-69
    average 92, 107
    high altitude 1
    isolated 40
    limited 25, 26
    major 15, 40
Nuclear disarmament 24
Nuclear power stations 89, 110
Nuclear radiation 9
Nuclear reactors 110
Nurses 40, 41
Nutrition 93, 123

Office block 74
Office of Technology Assessment (OTA) 47-78, 121
Oilwell 98
Openshaw, S. 22, 52-58, 70-79, 80, 89
Operational equivalent dose 86
Operational evaluation dose (OED) 86
Orthopaedic injuries 40
Overpressure 57-63, 77
Ozone 97, 98, 123

PIRC 84
Pain 42, 44
Paratyphoid 102
Pattern of attack 15, 56, 74, 121
Peace Movement 24
Peace time facilities 41, 42, 44, 92, 93
Penicillin 44
Permanent emergency footing 124
Personal health 100
Pertussis 102
Phosphine 44
Photochemical smog 98
Planning x, 110
Plant growth 98
Plants 96
Plasma 39, 44

Platelets 34, 42
Plutonium-239 2
Poliomyelitis 102
Population centres 74, 78, 120
Population density 57, 63, 120
Population distribution 56, 78
Population evacuation in USA 110
Power/fuel 40, 92, 122
Pre-emptive strike 121
Predicted casualties 81, 89
Pregnancy 43
'Protect and Survive' 52, 53, 75, 101
Protective factor 73-80
Protracted dose 83
Protracted radiation exposure 86
Psychiatric effect 37, 102
Psychological effects 35, 42, 108
Public health 100, 117, 123

Quinines 44

Rabies 102
Radiation
    carcinogenic effects 103
    long term effects 92, 103
Radiation doses 74, 77, 81, 87, 121
    brief exposure 85
Radiation erythema 34
Radiation injury 33
Radiation sickness 33, 36-50, 69
Radio and telecommunications 12, 14
Radioactive contamination 123
Radioactivity 39, 74, 77
Radiological recovery formula 86
'Refuge room' 75
Rehydration 101
Renal dialysis 108
Rescue Services 12, 39, 92
Rescue teams 38
Reservoirs 72
Residual radiation 6
Rheumatic fever 102
Rings (see Damage rings)
Rotblat, J. 7, 46, 77
Rural civilisation 123

SANA (see Scientists Against Nuclear Arms)
SIPRI (Stockholm International Peace Research Institute) 20-22
SS19 22
SS20 21, 22
SS4 21
SS5 21
Salt 101
Sanitation 35, 76, 104
Scientific advisers 22, 78
Scientists Against Nuclear Arms (SANA) 31, 48, 50, 121
Second World War (see World War II)
Sewers 9, 39, 72
Shelter period 77

Shelter pumps 109
Shelters 36, 40, 53, 62, 70, 74, 75, 76, 77, 108, 122
  Anderson 75
  commercial designs 75
  Home Office designs/Type 1, 2, 3, 4 75, 76, 77, 108
  Morrison 75
Shock 92
Shock wave 4, 5
Short term effects 34
Short term survival 82
Smog 98
Social disorganisation 36, 47
Sodium iodide 96
Solid tumours 103
Soviet weapons 17, 55
Special diets 108, 122
'Square Leg' 22, 40, 55, 58, 70, 73, 77, 78, 79
Steadman, P. 52-59, 63, 70, 73, 77-79, 80, 89
Steroid 44
Strategic weapons 17, 123
Stratosphere 99
Stress 35
Strokes 43
Strontium-90 96
Submarine launched ballistic missiles (SLBM) 17
Sulphonamide 44
Summerland Disaster 129
Surface tissue dose 88
Survival in shelters 108
Survivors 40, 45, 48, 62, 71, 96, 97, 100, 107, 114, 117
Synergistic injuries 45

TNT 8, 66
Tactical weapons 17, 26
Targets 15, 22, 45, 47, 56, 78, 120
Tension/political instability 17
Terms of reference x
Test-ban Treaty 62
Theatre weapons 17
Thermal radiation 4, 32, 45, 46, 58, 69, 70, 90
Thermonuclear bombs 6
Thoracic injuries 40
Three Mile Island 110
Thyroid cancer 103
Thyroid gland 96
Tissue damage (from radiation) 34, 35
Total killed 52, 65, 78
Tracy (Cyclone) 37
Transfusion (blood) 43, 44, 115
Trauma 41

Triage 38, 41
Tritium 7
Troposphere 99, 123
Tuberculosis 102
Typhoid 101, 102
Typhus 102

UK Medical Services 113, 123
US bases 21
US Department of Defense 62
USSR 17, 18, 20, 27
Uncertainty/imponderables 21, 46, 56, 121
Unique concentration of targets 22
United Kingdom 15, 21, 41, 67, 69, 74-85
United Nations 9, 31
United States 67, 78
Unreliability of basic assumptions 121
Uranium/Uranium-235 2

Vaccination 40
Vaccines 43
Vermin 96
Viral infections 102
Visibility 70
Volcanic dust 79
Voluntary Aid Societies 115
Voluntary organisations 116
Vomiting 33, 36, 42

WRVS 116
Warhead 9, 55
Warning period 19, 43, 70, 76
Water 39, 40, 44, 72, 76, 92, 122
  supplies 92, 122
  tanker 122
Weapons effects 46, 59
Weather 70, 71, 93
White cells (blood) 42
Whole body irradiation 42, 85
Wind 66, 73, 80
  direction 72, 73
  shear 6, 72
  speed 32, 72, 73
Windows (breaking of) 77, 80
World War II 37, 44, 66, 92, 102
Wound
  healing 84
  infection 39

X-rays xii, 7

Yield 15, 46, 57
Yield to weight ratio 8

Zuckerman 26, 27